Bone Grafting

Bone Grafting

Edited by **Shay Fisher**

hayle
medical

New York

Published by Hayle Medical,
30 West, 37th Street, Suite 612,
New York, NY 10018, USA
www.haylemedical.com

Bone Grafting
Edited by Shay Fisher

International Standard Book Number: 978-1-63241-060-3 (Hardback)

Printed in the United States of America.

Contents

Preface

The process of bone grafting has been explained in this book through descriptive information. Bone grafting is a surgical process in which a new bone or replacement material is inserted in bone fractures and bone defects in order to facilitate the process of repairing. It is of immense help even in cases which are tremendously complex, pose an important health risk to the patient, or fall short to heal correctly. Bone grafting holds an important place in variety of surgical specialties, such as: orthopedics, neurosurgery, dentistry, plastic surgery, neck and head surgery, otolaryngology and others. All these disciplines tackle problems related to absence of bone tissue or damaged fracture healing on a regular basis. A host of surgical techniques nowadays involve the use of one or other kind of bone graft or bone graft substitute. This book is a compilation of works of authors from different continents, with different perspectives and varied experiences with bone grafting. In this book, different readers can find reference content which suits their requisites. From basic principles, devoted to students, to research inferences and description of novel techniques, for experts; this book meets the needs of all those who are interested in the science of bone grafting.

Significant researches are present in this book. Intensive efforts have been employed by authors to make this book an outstanding discourse. This book contains the enlightening chapters which have been written on the basis of significant researches done by the experts.

Finally, I would also like to thank all the members involved in this book for being a team and meeting all the deadlines for the submission of their respective works. I would also like to thank my friends and family for being supportive in my efforts.

Editor

Part 1

Introduction

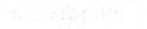

1

Introduction

Alessandro Rozim Zorzi and João Batista de Miranda
Campinas State University - UNICAMP,
Brazil

Bone grafting represents an exciting field of study and a major advance of modern surgery. It is an important tool that allows surgeons to deal with different and difficult situations. Massive tissue loss or impaired bone healing, caused by tumors, trauma, infections or congenital abnormalities, were unsolved problems until the recent development of bone grafting one century ago. Bone graft could be defined as a bone fragment transplanted, whole or in pieces, from one site to another. Bone grafting is the name of the surgical procedure, by which bone graft, or a bone graft substitute, is placed into fractures or bone defects, to aid in healing or to improve strength.

Bone is the second most commonly implanted material in the human body, after blood transfusion, with an estimated 600.000 grafts performed annually only in the USA [1].

Besides its frequent use, bone grafting study is also important because it is used by many specialties of Medicine and Dentistry, like Orthopedics, Traumatology, Neurosurgery, Spinal Surgery, Plastic Surgery, Hand Surgery, Head and Neck Surgery, Otolaryngology, Maxillofacial Surgery and others.

The correct and effective use of bone graft takes not only precise surgical technique skills, to harvest it and to deliver it to host bed, but also a deep theoretical knowledge, to understand its mechanical and biological behavior during graft integration to host tissues.

So, it is important to all surgeons and specialists involved somehow with bone grafting procedures, to have knowledge of some basic principles that will be presented along this and the following chapters. To understand the actual state of the art, it is important to begin by knowing the pioneers that initiate the history of bone grafting.

1.1 History

In the 19th century, three important scientific discoveries stimulated the rapid development of Modern Surgery: the advent of Anesthesia, attributed to William Thomas Green Morton in 1846; the use of asepsis and the development of an antiseptic solution to prevent infection in surgery, by Joseph Lister; the discovery of X-Ray by Wilhelm Conrad Röentegen, which performed the first radiography, taken by the hand of his wife in December 1895. These iscoveries boosted the surgical treatment of fractures during First World War [2].

Parallel to the rapid development of metallurgy, which allowed the rigid fixation of bone fractures with increasingly expensive implants, there was a slowly, but important, understanding of the biology of bone healing.

Although reports of autologous bone grafting date back to the ancient Egypt, the first description of systematic use of autologous bone grafting, with the modern principles and concepts, is attributed to **Fred H. Albee** (1876 – 1945), a North American surgeon that served during the First World War, and published in **1915** a textbook named **"Bone Graft Surgery"**. Before Albee, occasional reports described the use of various forms of bone grafts.

In the 17th century, there was an isolated report of a successful bone xenograft, performed by Job van Meekeren, who treated a bone defect in the skull of a Russian soldier with a dog's skull bone. It takes two centuries to appear a new reference about this kind of surgery. In 1881, MacEwen was able to reconstruct the umerus of a child with a cadaveric bone. Barth and Marchand also observed that the bone from autograft, when transplanted to another site, goes to necrosis and are subsequently invaded by host cells that differentiate to bone cells and produce new bone. In that way, those authors demonstrated that a fragment of bone take from one site can substitute bone from another site.

The French surgeon Léopold Ollier (1830-1900), called "The Father of Bone and Joint Surgery" and "The Father of Experimental Surgery", shed a significant light on the function of the periosteum, reflected in his "Traité de Régénération Osseuse Chez L'Animal". He also performed autologous and homologous bone grafting in humans.

Georg Axhausen (1877-1960) and Erich Lexer (1867-1937), German surgeons, and the North American surgeon Dallas B. Phemister (1882-1951), played an important role to make bone grafting recognized as rational and viable. Axhausen and Phemister described the graft incorporation process by the host organism. Lexer published clinical cases of bone allografting with twenty years follow-up, with good results in half of patients [3].

In the 40th decade, Wilson (1947) and Bush (1948) described freezing storage techniques for preserving allografts, giving rise to the era of tissue banking [4,5]. After the end of the Second World War, tissue banks become more complex, with the need to create protocols and rules to control the use and safety of musculoskeletal tissues. The American Association of Tissue Banks (AATB) was founded in 1976 by a group of doctors who had started in 1949 the first full tissue bank of the world, the United States Navy Tissue Bank [6].

Following the creation of AATB, the Asian Pacific Association of Surgical Tissue Banking was done. In a few years after 1949, additional regional tissue banks were established in Europe as well. Those first European regional and national tissue banks were established in the former Czechoslovakia in 1952, the former German Democratic Republic in 1956, in Great Britain 1955 and in Poland in 1962. Only after the end of the "Cold War" and the reunification of Berlin, it was born the European Association of Tissue Banks (EATB), in 1991 [7].

In the 60's decade, Marshall R Urist (1914-2001) established the osteoinductive capacity of Demineralized Bone Matrix (DBM), which leads to the discovering and understanding of a family of proteins called Bone Morphogenetic Proteins (BMPs) [8,9,10,11,12]. Both DBM and BMP are available nowadays to clinical use isolated or in combination with scaffolds. This finding started a new era in bone grafting, leading to the development of graft substitute research.

1.2 General indications for bone grafting

In brief, the major indications to the use of some kind of bone grafting procedure are the following [13]:

- Reconstruction of skeletal defects of multiple etiologies, like tumors, trauma, osteotomies and infections.
- Augmenting fracture healing, in the treatment of delayed-union and non-union, or in the prevention of those problems in patients with risk factors (smoking, diabetes).
- Fusing joints.
- Augmenting joint reconstruction procedures, especially to correct massive bone loss in revision arthroplasties.

1.3 Types of bone grafts

Bone grafts could be classified in different manners, according to its sources (table 1), surgical location (table 2) or time to use (table 3) [14,15].

Autograft	A graft moved from one site to another within the same individual.
Allograft	Tissue transferred between two genetically different individuals of the same species.
Xenograft	Tissue from one species into a member of a different species.
Isograft	Tissue from one twin implanted in an identical (monozygotic) twin.

Table 1. Type of bone graft according to its source.

Orthotopic	Anatomically appropriate site. Ex: delayed union of a bone fracture.
Heterotopic	Anatomically inappropriate site. Ex: subcutaneous tissue.

Table 2. Type of bone graft according to its surgical location.

Fresh	Transferred directly from the donor to the recipient site, in the case of autografts, or held for a relatively short time, in culture or storage medium, in the case of allografts (fresh-frozen).
Preserved	Maintained stored for a relatively long time in a tissue bank, by freezing, freeze-drying, irradiation or chemical treatment.

Table 3. Type of bone graft according to its time until implantation.

Bone grafts could also be classified as cortical, cancellous or corticocancellous, according to the type of bone present in the graft. Cortical bone grafts are used for structural support. Cancellous bone grafts are used for osteogenesis. These properties could be combined in a corticocancellous graft.

Although the name, vascularized bone grafts will not be approached in this chapter, because it is better understand in the field of microsurgical flaps.

1.4 Properties

Bone grafts present mechanical and biological properties. The biological properties are divided in Osteoconduction, Osteoinduction and Osteogenesis.

Osteoconduction is defined as the propertie of bone graft to serve as a framework to cells of the host (mature osteoblasts) that uses it as a porous three-dimensional scaffold to support in-growth. It depends of the host surrounding viable tissue to survive and incorporates. This effect could be exerted by autograft, allograft and bone graft substitutes. Autograft is always the gold-standard procedure; to wich the other must be compared. However, autograft harvest presents a series of complications, like pain, bloody loss, long surgical time, risk of nerve or vascular injurie, and scars. So the use of alternatives is very attractive, principally when the graft indication is for osteoconduction. Several artificial substitutes have been developed [16,17,18,19].

They could be divided in biological or non-biological materials.

Biological:

- Porous coralline ceramics
- Calcium sulfate
- Calcium phosphate
- Type 1 collagen (Col1);
- Numerous commercially available combinations of the above materials.

Non-biological:

- Degradable polymers (polylactic acid and polyglycolic acid);
- Bioactive glasses;
- Ceramics;
- Metals.

Osteoinduction is defined as the enhancement of bone formation, by the stimulation of host osteoprogenitor cells to differentiate to osteoblasts. It is used to enhance bone healing, to treat bone loss from trauma, tumor, osteonecrosis or congenital conditions. The gold-standard procedure is the autograft, but the pursuits of substitutes to avoid harvest complications lead to a significant improve in the understanding of growth factors that mediates bone formation. The most studied is a family of proteins called BMPs (Bone Morphogenetic Proteins).

Osteogenesis is defined as bone formation, from cells that survive in the graft and are capable of produce new bone. When new bone is formed from host cells which penetrate graft from surrounding tissue, this is called osteoinduction. It is indicated when the host conditions are impaired, like in fracture non-unions. Gold-standard procedure is autograft, but beyond the inconvenience of harvest, the limited quantity available is a major concern. With the development of tissue engineering, the combination of a scaffold with growth factors and stem cell derived osteo-progenitor cells has becoming a promissory field to provide large amounts of graft to fill large defects.

Mechanical properties are indicated to support weight-bearing. It could be exerted by autografts, like fibular non-vascularized transfer to support tibia bone loss (figure 1). With the development and expansion of the uses of joint arthroplasties, nowadays it is more common to use structural allografts in revision arthroplasty surgery to deal with large bone defects.

1.5 Sources of autollogous bone grafts

Surgeons must plan carefully any surgical procedure that involves bone grafting. Small amounts of cancellous grafts can be obtained from local sites nearby the surgical region:

- Greater trochanter of the femur for hip surgery;
- Femural condyle for knee surgery;
- Proximal tibial metaphysic for knee surgery;
- Medial malleolus of the tibia for ankle surgery;
- Olecranon for upper extremities;
- Distal radius for wrist surgery;

Large cancellous and corticocancellous grafts can be obtained from the anterosuperior iliac crest and the posterior iliac crest. Cancellous graft can be obtained also from the medular cavity when reaming procedures are performed.

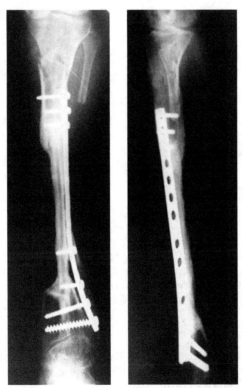

Fig. 1. An example of a structural autograft: after extensive bone loss caused by a high energy trauma, non-vascularized fibular diaphises was transferred to the tibia ("Tibialization of the Fibula") and fixed with plate and screws (pictures kindly provided by dr Bruno Livani).

1.6 Surgical techniques

1.6.1 Anterior iliac bone graft

If the patient is in the supine position for surgery, graft can be obtained from the anterosuperior iliac spine. This is a very dynamic source, as it provides cortical or cancellous grafts as well. If the intention is to use osteogenesis alone, bone chips can be removed. If mechanical support is required, a corticocancellous graft can be obtained with one, two or three cortical walls (figure 2).

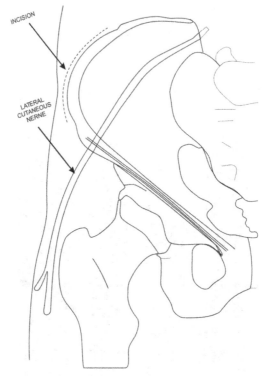

Fig. 2. Autologous bone graft could be obtained from the anterior region of the iliac bone. An oblique incision ("bikini incision") over the crest is performed carefully to avoid damage to the Lateral Thigh Cutaneous Nerve that runs medially to the Antero-Superior Iliac Spine, superficially to the Inguinal Ligament.

1.6.2 Posterior iliac bone graft

If the patient is prone, the posterior third of iliac bone is used. Caution should be taken to avoid Cluneal Nerves lesion, restricting the dissection to a line eight cm length from the posterior superior iliac spine (figure 3).

1.7 Complications of iliac autograft harvesting

- Bleeding and haematoma;

- Infection;
- Inguinal hernia;
- Nerve injury: the lateral femoral cutaneous and ilioinguinal nerves are at risk during anterior procedure. The superior cluneal nerves are at risk in the posterior procedure when dissection is extended beyond 8 cm lateral to posterosuperior iliac spine.
- Arterial injury: Superior gluteal vessels can be damaged by inadvertent retraction against the roof of sciatic notch. Arteriovenous fistula and pseudoaneurysm are less frequent.
- Cosmetic deformity;
- Pelvic fractures;
- Chronic pain;
- Insufficient material to fill the defect.

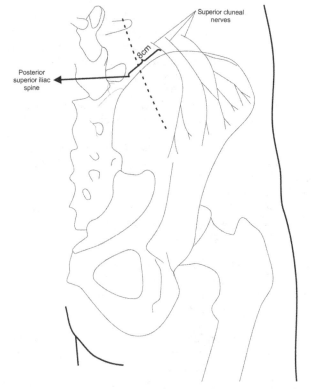

Fig. 3. To take bone from the posterior region of the iliac bone, a longitudinal incision is done crossing the iliac crest in a point between the Postero-Superior Iliac Spine and a point eight centimeters lateral to that, over the iliac crest, to avoid damage to the Cluneal nerves that runs in the subcutaneous tissue.

Nowadays, Autologous Bone Graft is the gold standard procedure. However, to avoid complications related to it, the pursuit of bone graft substitutes is one of the major fields in medical research today. The understanding of graft biology (osteogenesis, osteoinduction, osteoconduction) and integration to host tissue are paramount to the success of new materials. In the future, the developing of graft substitutes could be more safety and less expensive, turning the use of these materials the first choice when dealing with bone loss or fracture non-unions.

1.8 Acknowledgments

The authors would like to thank Dr. Bruno Livani (pictures) and Ms. Mercedes de Fátima Santos (illustrations design).

2. References

[1] Marino JT, Ziran BH."Use of solid and cancellous autologous bone graft for fractures and nonunions". Orthop Clin North Am.2010;41:15-26.
[2] The History of Medicine. Woods M, Woods MB. Twenty-First Century Books. 2006.
[3] Miranda JB. Regeneração do tecido ósseo esponjoso, em fêmures de cães, com auto-enxerto fragmentado e aloenxerto fragmentado e congelado [Thesis]. Campinas (SP):Universidade Estadual de Campinas;1996. Portuguese.
[4] Wilson PD."Experiences with a bone bank". Ann Surg.1947;126(6):932-46.
[5] Bush LF, Garber CZ."The bone bank".JAMA.1948;137(7):588-94.
[6] AATB.org [homepage on the internet]. McLean: American Association of Tissue Banks; c2010 [updated October 2011; cited October 22, 2011]. Available from: http://www.aatb.org.
[7] EATB.org [homepage on the internet]. Berlin: European Association of Tissue Banks; c2010 [updated January 2011; cited October 22, 2011]. Available from: http://www.eatb.org.
[8] Urist MR."Bone: formation by autoinduction".Science.1965;150(698):893-9.
[9] Urist MR, Silverman BF, Büring K, Dubuc FL, Rosenberg JM."The bone induction principle". Clin Orthop Relat Res.1967;53:243-83.
[10] Urist MR."The Classic: bone morphogenetic protein".Clin Orthop Relat Res. 2009;467(12):3051-62.
[11] Nogami H, Urist MR."The Classic: a morphogenic matrix for differentiation of cartilage in tissue culture". Clin Orthop Relat Res.2009;467(12):3063-7.
[12] Urist MR."The Classic: a morphogenic matrix for differentiation of bone tissue". Clin Orthop Relat Res.2009;467(12):3068-70.
[13] Campbell's Operative Orthopedics. S. Therry Canale. 10ª Edtion. Mosby 2003.
[14] Stevenson S."Biology of bone grafts". Orthop Clin North Am.1999;30(4):543-52.
[15] Stevenson S."Enhancement of fracture healing with autogenous and allogeneic bone grafts". Clin Orthop Relat Res.1998;355S:S239-S246.
[16] Cornell CN."Osteoconductive materials and their role as substitutes for autogenous bone grafts". Orthop Clin North Am.1999;30(4):591-8.
[17] Sanders R."Bone graft substitutes: separating fact from fiction". J Bone J Surg (Am).2007;89A(3):469.
[18] De Long Jr WG, Einhorn TA, Koval K, McKee M, Watson T, et al."Bone grafts and bone graft substitutes in orthopaedic trauma surgery". J Bone J Surg Am.2007;89A(3):649-58.
[19] Giannoudis PV, Dinopoulos H, Tsiridis E."Bone substitutes: an update". Injury. 2005;36S:S20-7.

2

Basic Knowledge of Bone Grafting

Nguyen Ngoc Hung
Hanoi Medial University,
Military Academy of Medicine,
Pediatric Orthopaedic Department - National Hospital of Pediatrics,
Dong Da District, Ha Noi,
Vietnam

1. Introduction

Bone grafting is a surgical procedure that replaces missing bone in order bone fractures that are extremely complex, pose a significant health risk to the patient, or fail to heal property.

Bone grafting is a very old surgical procedure. The first recorded bone implant was performed in 1668. Bone grafts are used to treat various disorders, including delayed union and nonunion of fractures, congenital pseudoarthrosis, and osseous defects from trauma, infection, and tumors. Bone grafts are also used in plastic and facial surgery for reconstruction.

Bone generally has the ability to regenerate completely but requires a very small fracture space or some sort of scaffold to do so. Bone grafts may be autogous (bone harvested from the patient's own body, often from iliac crest), allograft (cadaveric bone usually obtained from a bone bank), or synthetic (often made of hydroxyapatite or other naturally occurring and biocompatible substances) with similar mechanical properties to bone. Most bone grafts are expeted to be reabsorbed and replaced as the natural bone heals over a few month's time.

The principles, indications, and techniques of bone grafting procedures were well established before "the metallurgic age" of orthopaedic surgery. Because of the necessity of using autogenous materials such as bone pegs or, in some cases, using wire loops, fixation of grafts was rather crude. Lane and Sandhu introduced internal fixation; Albee and Kushner, Henderson, Campbell, and others added osteogenesis to this principle to develop bone grafting for nonunion into a practical procedure. The two principles, fixation and osteogenesis, were not, however, efficiently and simply combined until surgeons began osseous fixation with inert metal screws. Then came the bone bank with its obvious advantages. Much work, both clinical and experimental, is being done to improve the safety and results of bone grafting: donors are being more carefully selected to prevent the transmission of HIV and other diseases; tissue typing and the use of immunosuppressants are being tried; autologous bone marrow is being added to autogenous and homogenous bone grafts to stimulate osteogenesis; and bone graft substitutes have been developed.

Bone graft are involved in successful bone graft include osteoconduction (guiding the reparative growth of the natural bone), osteoinduction (encouraging undifferentiated cells to become active osteoblast), and osteogenesis (living bone cells in the graft material contribute to become remodeling). Osteogenesis only occurs with autografts.

Bone grafts may be used for the following purposes:

1. To fill cavities or defects resulting from cysts, tumors, or other causes
2. To bridge joints and thereby provide arthrodesis
3. To bridge major defects or establish the continuity of a long bone
4. To provide bone blocks to limit joint motion (arthrorisis)
5. To establish union in a pseudarthrosis
6. To promote union or fill defects in delayed union, malunion, fresh fractures, or osteotomies
7. To plastical arthrosis of acetabulum for Congenital Dislocation of the Hip and Perthes disease

2. Basic knowledge of bone grafting

Phemister introduced the term creeping substitution [1, 2]. He believed that transplanted bone was invaded by vascular granulation tissue, causing the old bone to be resorbed and subsequently replaced by the host with new bone. Phemister's concept remains valid; however, Abbott and associates have shown that, in addition, surface cells in the bone graft survive and participate in new bone formation [3]. Ray and Sabet [4] and Arora and Laskin [5] also confirmed the fact that superficial cells in the bone graft probably survive transplantation and contribute to new bone formation. The percentage of cells that survive transplantation is unknown, but cell survival seems to be improved by minimizing the interval between harvest and implantation and by keeping the graft moist and at physiologic temperatures.

In cancellous bone grafts, the necrotic tissue in marrow spaces and haversian canals is removed by macrophages. Granulation tissue, preceded by the advance of capillaries, invades the areas of resorption [6]. Pluripotential mesenchymal cells differentiate into osteoblasts, which begin to lay seams of osteoid along the dead trabeculae of the bone graft. Osteoclasts resorb the necrotic bone, and eventually most of the bone graft is replaced by new host bone. Finally, the old marrow space is filled by new marrow cells [7].

In cortical bone, the process of incorporation is similar but much slower, because invasion of the graft must be through the haversian canals of the transplant [8]. Osteoclasts resorb the surface of the canals, creating larger spaces into which granulation tissue grows. As this granulation tissue penetrates the center of the cortical graft, new bone is laid throughout the graft along enlarged haversian canals. Depending on the size of the graft, complete replacement may take many months to a year or more [9].

2.1 Biological mechanism

Osteoconduction

Osteoconduction occurs when the bone graft material serves as a scaffold for new bone growth that is perpetuated by the native bone. Osteoblasts from the margin of the defect that is being grafted utilize the bone graft material as a framework upon which to spread and generate new bone. In the very least, a bone graft material should be osteoconductive.

Osteoinduction

Osteoinduction involves the stimulation of osteoprogenitor cells to differentiate into osteoblasts that then begin new bone formation. The most widely studied type of osteoinductive cell mediators are bone morphogenetic proteins (BMPs). A bone graft material that is osteoconductive and osteoinductive will not only serve as a scaffold for currently existing osteoblasts but will also trigger the formation of new osteoblasts, theoretically promoting faster integration of the graft.

Osteogenesis

Osteogenesis occurs when vital osteoblasts originating from the bone graft material contribute to new bone growth along with bone growth generated via the other two mechanisms.

Osteopromotion

Osteopromotion involves the enhancement of osteoinduction without the possession of osteoinductive properties. For example, enamel matrix derivative has been shown to enhance the osteoinductive effect of demineralized freeze dried bone allograft (DFDBA), but will not stimulate denovo bone growth alone [3].

2.2 Structure of grafts

Cortical bone grafts are used primarily for structural support, and cancellous bone grafts for osteogenesis. Structural support and osteogenesis may be combined; this is one of the prime advantages of using bone graft. These two factors, however, vary with the structure of the bone. Probably all or most of the cellular elements in grafts (particularly cortical grafts) die and are slowly replaced by creeping substitution, the graft merely acting as a scaffold for the formation of new bone. In hard cortical bone this process of replacement is considerably slower than in spongy or cancellous bone. Although cancellous bone is more osteogenic, it is not strong enough to provide efficient structural support. When selecting the graft or combination of grafts, the surgeon must be aware of these two fundamental differences in bone structure. Once a graft has united with the host and is strong enough to permit unprotected use of the part, remodeling of the bone structure takes place commensurate with functional demands.

Bone grafts may be cortical, cancellous, or corticocancellous. If structural strength is required, cortical bone grafts must be used. However, the process of replacement produces resorption as early as 6 weeks after implantation; in dogs, it may take up to 1 year before the graft begins to regain its original mechanical strength [10]. Drilling holes in the graft does not appear to accelerate the process of repair, but it may lead to the early formation of biologic pegs that enhance graft union to host bone [11].

2.3 Sources of grafts

Bone graft terminology has changed, leading to some confusion. In this text, we use the new terminology. For most applications, autogenous bone graft is indicated. Other types of bone grafts are indicated only if autogenous bone graft is unavailable or if it is insufficient and must be augmented. Another exception is when structural whole or partial bones, with or without joint articular surfaces, are needed for reconstruction of massive whole or partial bone defects [12 - 15].

Autogenous grafts, when the bone grafts come from the patient, the grafts usually are removed from the tibia, fibula, or ilium. These three bones provide cortical grafts, whole bone transplants, and cancellous bone, respectively.

When internal or external fixation appliances are not used, which is rare now, strength is necessary in a graft used for bridging a defect in a long bone or even for the treatment of pseudarthrosis. The subcutaneous anteromedial aspect of the tibia is an excellent source for such grafts. In adults, after removal of a cortical graft, the plateau of the tibia supplies cancellous bone. Apparently, leaving the periosteum attached to the graft has no advantage; however, suturing to the periosteum over the defect has definite advantages.

3. Type and tissue sources

3.1 Autograft

Autologous (or autogenous) bone grafting involves utilizing bone obtained from the same individual receiving the graft.

When a block graft will be performed, autogenous bone is the most preferred because there is less risk of the graft rejection because the graft originated from the patient's own body [16]. As indicated in the chart above, such a graft would be osteoinductive and osteogenic, as well as osteoconductive. A negative aspect of autologous grafts is that an additional surgical site is required, in effect adding another potential location for post-operative pain and complications [17].

All bone requires a blood supply in the transplanted site. Depending on where the transplant site and the size of the graft, an additional blood supply may be required. For these types of grafts, extraction of the part of the periosteum and accompanying blood vesels along with donor bone is required. This kind of graft is known as a vital bone graft.

An autograft may also be performed without a solid bony structure, for example using bone reamed from the anterior superior iliac spine. In this case there is an osteoinductive and osteogenic action, however there is no osteoconductive action, as there is no solid bony structure.

3.2 Allografts

Allograft bone, like autogenous bone, is derived from humans; the difference is that allograft is harvested from an individual other than the one receiving the graft. Allograft bone is taken from cadavers that have donated their bone so that it can be used for living people who are in need of it; it is typically sourced from a bone bank.

In small children the usual donor sites do not provide cortical grafts large enough to bridge defects, or the available cancellous bone may not be enough to fill a large cavity or cyst; furthermore, the possibility of injuring a physis must be considered. Therefore grafts for small children usually were removed from the father or mother.

Heterogeneous Grafts. Because of the undesirable features of autogenous and allogenic bone grafting, heterogenous bone, that is, bone from another species, was tried early in the development of bone grafting and was found to be almost always unsatisfactory. The material more or less retained its original form, acting as an internal splint but not stimulating bone production. These grafts often incited an undesirable foreign body reaction. Consistently satisfactory heterogenous graft material still is not commercially available, and its use is not recommended.

Cancellous Bone Substitutes. Hydroxyapatite and tricalcium phosphate, synthetic and naturally occurring materials, are now being used as substitutes for cancellous bone grafts in certain circumstances. These porous materials are invaded by blood vessels and osteogenic cells, provide a scaffold for new bone formation, and are, in theory, eventually replaced by bone. Their primary usefulness is in filling cancellous defects in areas where graft strength is not important. Bucholz et al. found hydroxyapatite and tricalcium phosphate materials to be effective alternatives to autogenous cancellous grafts for grafting tibial plateau fractures. A synthetic bone graft substitute composed of biphasic ceramic (60% hydroxyapatite and 40% tricalcium phosphate) plus type I bovine collagen and marketed as Collagraft (Zimmer, Warsaw, Ind.) has recently undergone clinical trials.

3.3 Synthetic variants

Artificial bone can be created from ceramics such as calcium phosphates (e.g. hydroxyapatite and tricalcium phosphate), Bioglass and calcium sulphate; all of which are biologically active to different degrees depending on solubility in the physiological environment [18]. These materials can be doped with growth factors, ions such as strontium or mixed with bone marrow aspirate to increase biological activity. Some authors believe this method is inferior to autogenous bone grafting [16] however infection and rejection of the graft is much less of a risk, the mechanical properties such as Young's modulus are comparable to bone.

3.4 Xenografts

Xenograft bone substitute has its origin from a species other than human, such as bovine. Xenografts are usually only distributed as a calcified matrix. In January 2010 Italian scientists announced a breakthrough in the use of wood as a bone substitute, though this technique is not expected to be used for humans until at the earliest [19]

3.5 Alloplastic grafts

Alloplastic grafts may be made from hydroxylapatite, a naturally occurring mineral that is also the main mineral component of bone. They may be made from bioactive glass. Hydroxylapetite is a Synthetic Bone Graft, which is the most used now among other synthetic due to its osteoconduction, hardness and acceptability by bone. Some synthetic bone grafts are made of calcium carbonate, which start to decrease in usage because it is completely resorbable in short time which make the bone easy to break again. Finally used is the tricalcium phosphate which now used in combination with hydroxylapatite thus give both effect osteoconduction and resorbability.

3.6 Bone bank

Opinions differ among orthopaedic surgeons regarding the use of preserved allogenic bone, although its practical advantages are many. Fresh autogenous bone must generally be obtained through a second incision, which adds to the size and length of the operation and to the blood loss. After removal of a cortical graft from the tibia, the leg must be protected to prevent fracture at the donor site. At times it is not possible to obtain enough autogenous bone to meet the needs of the operation.

If osteogenesis is the prime concern, fresh autogenous bone is the best graft. Autogenous bone is preferable when grafting nonunions of fractures of the long bones. If stability is not required of a graft, cancellous autogenous iliac grafts are superior to autogenous grafts from the tibia. Allografts are indicated in small children, aged persons, patients who are poor operative risks, and patients from whom enough acceptable autogenous bone is not available. Autogenous cancellous bone can be mixed in small amounts with allograft bone as "seed" to provide osteogenic potential. Mixed bone grafts of this type will incorporate more rapidly than allograft bone alone.

To efficiently provide safe and useful allograft material, a bone banking system is required that uses thorough donor screening, rapid procurement, and safe, sterile processing. Standards outlined by the American Association of Tissue Banks must be followed. Donors must be screened for bacterial, viral (including HIV and hepatitis), and fungal infection. Malignancy (except basal cell carcinoma of the skin), collagen-vascular disease, metabolic bone disease, and the presence of toxins are all contraindications to donation.

Nearly one third of all bone grafts used in North America are allografts [18]. Allografts have osteoconductive proprieties and can serve as substitutes for autografts but carry the risk of disease transmission. The risk for transmission of human immunodeficiency virus (HIV) is 1:1,500,000; for hepatitis C, the risk is 1:60,000; and for hepatitis B, it is 1:100,000 [17].

The U.S. Food and Drug Administration (FDA) requires testing for HIV-1, HIV-2, and hepatitis C; many states require additional testing for hepatitis B core antibody [5] The American Association of Tissue Banks additionally tests for antibodies to human T-cell lymphotrophic virus (HTLV-I and HTLV-II) [18].

4. Growth factors

Growth Factor enhanced grafts are produced using recombinant DNA technology. They consist of either Human Growth Factors or Morphogens (Bone Morphogenic Proteins in conjunction with a carrier medium, such as collagen).

5. Position of bone grafting is harvested

5.1 Sources of cancellous bone

In treating small bone defects secondary to trauma or small tumors, it may be most convenient to harvest the graft from the ipsilateral extremity undergoing operation. The graft can often be taken through the same incision or through a small, separate incision. Most of these sites can be harvested through a small, 2.5 to 5.0 cm longitudinal incision placed over the subcutaneous surface of the end.

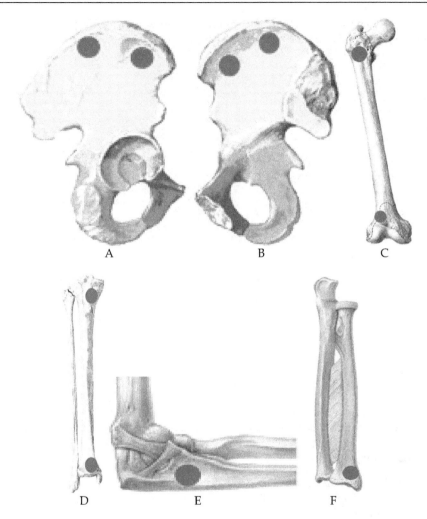

● Donor site

Fig. 1. Peripheral sources of cancellous bone graft are illustrated. If only a small amount of cancellous bone is needed or if it is contraindicated or inconvenient to use the iliac crest, other sites of cancellous bone are the anterior aspect of the greater trochanter and the distal femoral condyle (C), the proximal and distal tibia (D), the olecranon (E), and the styloid of the radius (F).

5.2 Removal of tibial graft

Make a slightly curved longitudinal incision over the anteromedial surface of the tibia, placing it so as to prevent a painful scar over the crest. Because of the shape of the tibia, the graft is usually wider at the proximal end than at the distal [20]. The periosteum over the tibia is relatively thick in children and can usually be sutured as a separate layer. In adults, however, it is often thin, and closure may be unsatisfactory; suturing the periosteum and the deep portion of the subcutaneous tissues as a single layer is usually wise.

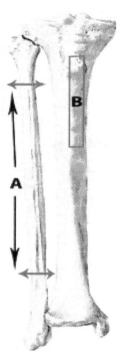

Fig. 2. A – Fibula can be harvested longitudinal bone; B- tibial graft is shown: a large, corticocancellous graft can be removed from the proximal tibia on its anteromedial surface.

5.3 Removal of fibular graft

In the removal of a fibular graft three points should receive consideration: (1) the peroneal nerve must not be damaged; (2) the distal fourth of the bone must be left to maintain a stable ankle; and (3) the peroneal muscles should not be cut.

The entire proximal two thirds of the fibula may be removed without materially disabling the leg. However, a study by Gore et al. indicates that most patients have complaints and mild muscular weakness after removal of a portion of the fibula. The configuration of the proximal end of the fibula is an advantage: the proximal end has a rounded prominence, which is partially covered by hyaline cartilage, and thus forms a satisfactory transplant to replace the distal third of the radius or the distal third of the fibula.

The middle one third of the fibula also can be used as a vascularized free autograft based on the peroneal artery and vein pedicle using microvascular technique. This graft is recommended by Simonis, Shirall, and Mayou for the treatment of large defects in congenital pseudarthrosis of the tibia. Portions of iliac crest also can be used as free vascularized autograft. The use of free vascularized autografts has limited indications, requires expert microvascular technique, and is not without donor site morbidity.

5.4 Removal of iliac bone graft

Ilium

The iliac crest is an ideal source of bone graft because it is relatively subcutaneous, has natural curvatures that are useful in fashioning grafts, has ample cancellous bone, and has cortical bone of varying thickness. Removal of the bone carries minimal risk and usually there is no significant residual disability. The posterior third of the ilium is thickest, and this is confirmed by computer tomography (CT) scans (Fig. 3).

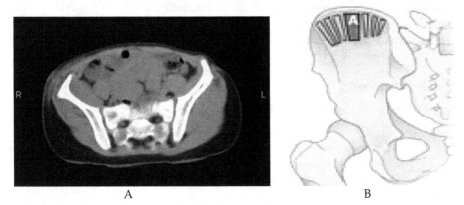

A   B

Fig. 3. A: This CT scan of the pelvis at the level of the posterosuperior iliac spine illustrates the thickness of the ilium posteriorly and the amount of cancellous bone available; B: The central section of the ilium at point A is quite thin and is of no use in bone grafting

5.5 Cancellous grafts

Unless considerable strength is required, the cancellous graft fulfills almost any requirement. Regardless of whether the cells in the graft remain viable, clinical results indicate that cancellous grafts incorporate with the host bone more rapidly than do cortical grafts.

Large cancellous and corticocancellous grafts may be obtained from the anterosuperior iliac crest and the posterior iliac crest. Small cancellous grafts may be obtained from the greater trochanter of the femur, femoral condyle, proximal tibial metaphysis, medial malleolus of the tibia, olecranon, and distal radius. At least 2 cm of subchondral bone must remain to avoid collapse of the articular surface.

5.6 Removal of iliac bone graft

When removing a cortical graft from the outer table, first outline the area with an osteotome or power saw. Then peel the graft up by slight prying motions with a broad osteotome.

Wedge grafts or full-thickness grafts may be removed more easily with a power saw; this technique also is less traumatic than when an osteotome and mallet are used. For this purpose an oscillating saw or an air-powered cutting drill is satisfactory. Avoid excessive heat by irrigating with saline at room temperature. Avoid removing too much of the crest anteriorly and leaving an unsightly deformity posteriorly (Figure 4).

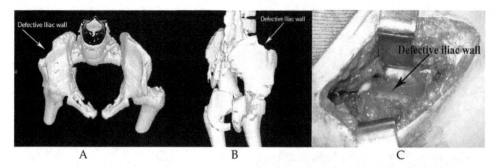

Fig. 4. A: CT scan 3D, Anteroposterior ilium and CT scan 3D, B: oblique posterior ilium with defect in iliac wall after iliac bone is harvested; C: The Iliac wall with defect.

5.7 Posterior iliac grafts

The region of the posterosuperior iliac spine is the best source of cancellous bone.

-   Make a straight vertical incision directly over the posterosuperior iliac spine or a curvilinear incision that parallels the iliac crest (Fig. 5). To prevent injury to the cluneal nerves, avoid straight transverse incisions and try not to carry incisions too far laterally. A transverse incision is more likely to result in dehiscence and can be painful if it lies along the belt line.
-   Identify the origin and fascia of the gluteus maximus insertion on the crest. With a cautery knife, incise the origin of the gluteus maximus and dissect it free from the crest subperiosteally. If the entire posterior iliac area is to be harvested, take down the gluteus from approximately 2.5 cm superior to the posterosuperior iliac spine and inferior as far as the posteroinferior spine.
-   The outer wall of the ilium is removed by first outlining the area to be harvested by cutting through the outer table of the ilium with a sharp osteotome. If an onlay cancellous bone graft is to be performed, harvest corticocancellous strips with a curved gouge. Remove all underlying cancellous bone down to the inner table of the ilium with a curved gouge and curets of an appropriate size.

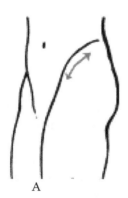
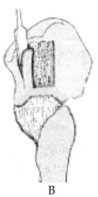

Fig. 5. A: Incision line; B: posterior iliac graft is shown.

5.8 Anterior iliac grafts

Large grafts of cancellous and corticocancellous bone can be harvested from the anterior ilium.

Incise with a cautery knife along the iliac crest, avoiding muscle. Subperiosteally, dissect the abdominal musculature and, subsequently, the iliacus from the inner wall of the ilium.

- Outline the area to be harvested with straight and curved osteotomes. Cut the strips, which will be removed. The middle ilium is paper thin, but the anterior column just above the acetabulum is quite thick.
- Harvest the corticocancellous strips with a gouge.
- Remove additional cancellous bone with gouges and curets. Do not broach the outer table.

5.9 Bicortical grafts

Full-thickness bicortical grafts may be necessary for spinal fusion or for replacement of major bone defects in metaphyseal regions, such as in nonunions of the distal humerus or in opening wedge osteotomies.

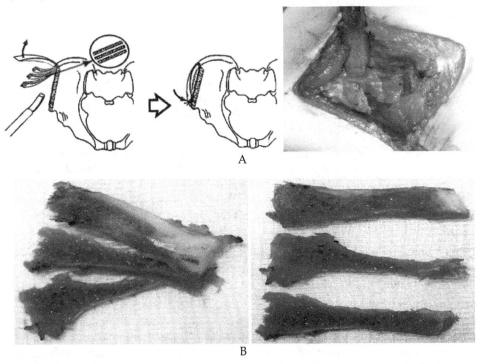

Fig. 6. A and B: Thin bicorticalcancellous grafts is harvested for Congenital pseudarthrosis of the tibia (From Author - Hung NN. Use of an intramedullary Kirschner wire for treatment of congenital pseudarthrosis of the tibia in children. Journal of Pediatric Orthopaedics B 2009; 18:79–85 [21])

6. Practical bone grafting

6.1 Bone grafting fundamentals

Bone grafting refers to a wide variety of surgical methods augmenting or stimulating the formation of new bone where it is needed.

There are five broad clinical situations in which bone grafting is performed:

1. To stimulate healing of fractures either fresh fractures or fractures that have failed to heal after an initial treatment attempt.
2. To stimulate healing between two bones across a diseased joint. This situation is called "arthrodesis" or "fusion".
3. To regenerate bone which is lost or missing as a result of trauma, infection, or disease. Settings requiring reconstruction or repair of missing bone can vary from filling small cavities to replacing large segments of bone 12 or more inches in length.
4. To improve the bone healing response and regeneration of bone tissue around surgically implanted devices, such as artificial joints replacements (e.g. total hip replacement or total knee replacement) or plates and screws used to hold bone alignment.
5. To plastical arthrosis of acetabulum (Congenital Dislocation of the Hip or Perthes disease)

6.2 Indications for various techniques

Single Onlay Cortical Grafts. Until relatively inert metals became available, the onlay bone graft was the simplest and most effective treatment for most ununited diaphyseal fractures. Usually the cortical graft was supplemented by cancellous bone for osteogenesis. The onlay graft is still applicable to a limited group of fresh, malunited, and ununited fractures and after osteotomies.

Cortical grafts also are used when bridging joints to produce arthrodesis, not only for osteogenesis but also for fixation. Fixation as a rule is best furnished by internal or external metallic devices. Only in an extremely unusual situation would a cortical onlay graft be indicated for fixation, and then only in small bones and when little stress is expected. For osteogenesis the thick cortical graft has largely been replaced by thin cortical and cancellous bone from the ilium.

The single-onlay cortical bone graft was used most commonly before the development of good quality internal fixation and was employed for both osteogenesis and fixation in the treatment of nonunions (Fig. 7).

Dual Onlay Grafts. Dual onlay bone grafts are useful when treating difficult and unusual nonunions or for the bridging of massive defects. The treatment of a nonunion near a joint is difficult, since the fragment nearest the joint is usually small, osteoporotic, and largely cancellous, having only a thin cortex. It is often so small and soft that fixation with a single graft is impossible because screws tend to pull out of it and wire sutures cut through it. Dual grafts provide stability because they grip the small fragment like forceps.

The advantages of dual grafts for bridging defects are as follows: (1) mechanical fixation is better than fixation by a single onlay bone graft; (2) the two grafts add strength and stability;

(3) the grafts form a trough into which cancellous bone may be packed; and (4) during healing the dual grafts, unlike a single graft, prevent contracting fibrous tissue from compromising transplanted cancellous bone.

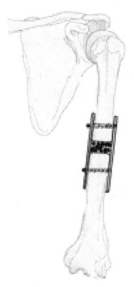

Fig. 7. A single-onlay cortical bone graft is shown for humeral pseudarthrose.

The disadvantages of dual grafts are the same as those of single cortical grafts: (1) they are not as strong as metallic fixation devices; (2) an extremity must usually serve as a donor site if autogenous grafts are used; and (3) they are not as osteogenic as autogenous iliac grafts, and the surgery necessary to obtain them has more risk.

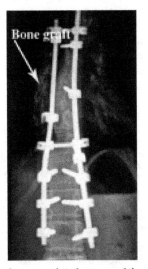

Fig. 8. Cortical cortical cancellous bone graft is harvested from Ilium for scoliosis

Inlay Grafts. By the inlay technique a slot or rectangular defect is created in the cortex of the host bone, usually with a power saw. A graft the same size or slightly smaller is then fitted into the defect. In the treatment of diaphyseal nonunions, the onlay technique is simpler and more efficient and has almost replaced the inlay graft. The latter is still occasionally used in arthrodesis, particularly at the ankle.

Albee popularized the inlay bone graft for the treatment of nonunions [22, 23]. Inlay grafts are created by a sliding technique, graft reversal technique, or as a strut graft. Although originally designed for the treatment of nonunion of the tibia, these techniques are also used for arthrodesis and epiphyseal arrest.

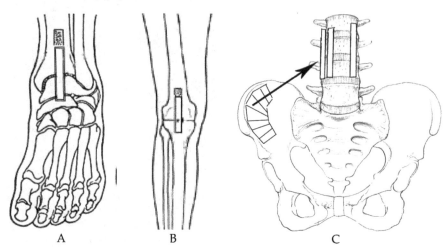

A   B   C

Fig. 9. A-C. A: In this case, a sliding graft is used as a component of ankle arthrodesis. This type of graft is more likely to be used for a previously failed ankle fusion or for fusion in the absence of the body of the talus; B: a sliding graft is used as a component of knee arthrodesis. This type of graft is more likely to be used for a previously failed knee fusion; C: Strut grafts for anterior spinal fusion. Strut grafts are very useful for bridging defects in the anterior spine and for providing support for anterior spinal fusion. Grafts from the ribs, fibula, and bicortical iliac crest are useful for strut grafting, depending on the size of the graft needed.

Dormans et al. reviewed their experience with the treatment of fourteen children who had osteoblastoma. The mean age at the time of diagnosis was nine years, and the lesions were most frequently seen in the lower extremities (43%) or the spine (36%). The patients were treated with open incisional biopsy and intralesional curettage, and those with a spinal lesion were also treated with spinal fusion and instrumentation. The local recurrence rate was 28%, and all recurrences were in young children who were less than six years of age.

7. Tumor

Medullary Grafts. Medullary bone grafts were tried early in the development of bone grafting techniques for nonunion of the diaphyseal fractures. Fixation was insecure, and healing was rarely satisfactory. This graft interferes with endosteal circulation and consequently can interfere with healing.

Medullary grafts are not indicated for the diaphysis of major long bones. Grafts in this location interfere with restoration of endosteal blood supply; because they are in the central axis of the bone, they resorb rather than incorporate. The only possible use for a medullary graft is in the metacarpals and the metatarsals, where the small size of the bone enhances incorporation. Even in this location, however, internal fixation with onlay or intercalary cancellous bone grafting may be a superior method.

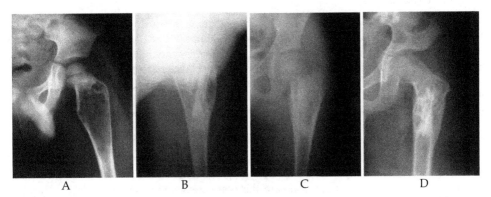

Fig. 10. A – D. A: Anteroposterior radiographs show an Giant cell tumor in proximal femur of 7-year-old child. B: the cavity of the proximal femur after curettage and the fibula strut autograft in cavity and the cavity is completely packed with particulate autograft around the fibula strut; C: Eight month after operation; D: Twenty-six months after operation, remodeling of bone tissue is evident.

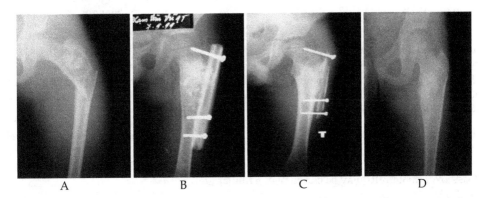

Fig. 11. A - D. A: Anteroposterior radiographs show an osteoblastoma with an associated aneurysmal bone cyst and pathology fracture in the neck and proximal femu; B: the cavity of the neck and proximal femur after curettage and the fibula strut allograft in lateral femur, the cavity is shown after being completely packed with particulate bone graft; C: Anteroposterior radiographs show postoperative result 28 months; D: Roentgenogram at 9 years follow-up showing incorporation of graft, remodeling, and full range of motion of hip joint.

7.1 Osteoperiosteal grafts

In osteoperiosteal grafts, the periosteum is harvested with chips of cortical bone. These grafts have not been proven to be superior to onlay cancellous bone grafting, are more difficult than cancellous bone to harvest, and may involve greater morbidity; they are rarely used today.

7.2 Pedicle grafts

Pedicle grafts may be local [24] or moved from a remote site using microvascular surgical techniques. In local muscle-pedicle bone grafts, an attempt is made to preserve the viability of the graft by maintaining muscle and ligament attachments carrying blood supply to the bone or, in the case of diaphyseal bone, by maintaining the nutrient artery. Two examples are the transfer of the anterior iliac crest on the muscle attachments of the sartorius and rectus femoris for use in the Davis type of hip fusion and the transfer of the posterior portion of the greater trochanter on a quadratus muscle pedicle for nonunions of the femoral neck [25-27].

Osteoperiosteal Grafts. Osteoperiosteal grafts are less osteogenic than multiple cancellous grafts and are now rarely used.

Multiple Cancellous Chip Grafts. Multiple chips of cancellous bone are widely used for grafting. Segments of cancellous bone are the best osteogenic material available. They are particularly useful for filling cavities or defects resulting from cysts, tumors, or other causes, for establishing bone blocks, and for wedging in osteotomies. Being soft and friable, this bone can be packed into any nook or crevice. The ilium is a good source of cancellous bone, and if some rigidity and strength are desired, the cortical elements may be retained.

In most bone-grafting procedures that use cortical bone or metallic devices for fixation, supplementary cancellous bone chips or strips are used to hasten healing. Cancellous grafts are particularly applicable to arthrodesis of the spine, since osteogenesis is the prime concern [28].

Hemicylindrical Grafts. Hemicylindrical grafts are suitable for obliterating large defects of the tibia and femur. A massive hemicylindrical cortical graft from the affected bone is placed across the defect and is supplemented by cancellous iliac bone. A procedure of this magnitude has only limited use, but it is applicable for resection of bone tumors when amputation is to be avoided.

The fibula provides the most practical graft for bridging long defects in the diaphyseal portion of bones of the upper extremity, unless the nonunion is near a joint. A fibular graft is stronger than a full-thickness tibial graft, and when soft tissue is a wound that could not be closed over dual grafts may be closed over a fibular graft.

7.3 Sliding graft

This technique is rarely used today, because internal fixation combined with onlay cancellous bone graft provides a better result. This technique may be combined with internal fixation if there is limited space to place a cancellous graft. The disadvantages of the sliding or reversed bone graft are that, after the cuts are made, the graft fits loosely in the bed, and it creates stress risers proximally and distally to the nonunion site

7.4 Peg and Dowel grafts

Dowel grafts were developed for the grafting of nonunions in anatomic areas, such as the scaphoid and femoral neck, where onlay bone grafting was impractical. In the carpal scaphoid, the dowel is fashioned from dense cancellous bone. The use of the dowel graft for the management of nonunion of the femoral neck. Free microvascularized fibula grafts are more commonly used today. A corticocancellous graft of appropriate length and approximately 25 mm wide is harvested from the ilium or the tibia. The curvature of the ilium often makes it difficult to obtain a straight graft of sufficient length.

7.5 Fibular bone gafting for defect of tibia cause osteomyelitis

The rules of bone grafting for long defects in the diaphyseal portion of extremity due to osteomyelitis are: (1). General status is stable: ESR: < 10 mm/h; CRP: < 10 mg/L ; WBC: < 10.000; Neutrophil: < 60%; (2) Local extremity with bone defect: no swelling, no hot-temperature, no pain, and no pus fistula for at least 3 months; (3) Remove sclerosis bone until bone bleeding; (4) Solid fixation of bone graft into bone bed by Kirschner wire or plate and screw and plaste cast ; (5) The Kirschner wire will be removed when clear clinical and radiographic evidence of solid union were apparent (mean more than 18 months); and (6) Prolonged orthotic protection was required when ankle transfixation had been performed and A knee-ankle-foot orthosis was worn until the patient reached skeletal maturity.

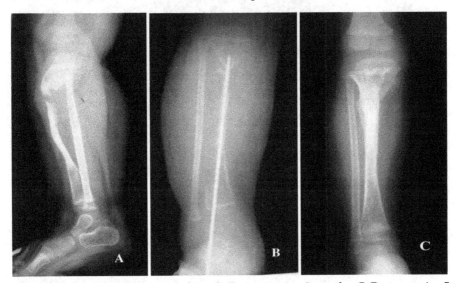

Fig. 16. A-C: A: Preoperative bone grafting; B: Postoperative 6 months; C: Postoperative 5 years 9 months.

7.6 Dual-onlay cortical cancellous bone graft is harvested Ilium for congenital pseudarthrosis of the tibia

The rules of bone grafting for Congenital Tibial Pseudarthrosis: (1) The bone and fibrous tissue at the site of the pseudarthrosis are excised completely until normal bone of the tibial shaft; (2) The medullary canal of both tibial fragments is reamed with a drill or a small curet, or both; (3) The autogenous iliac crest bone graft was applied to anterolateral and posterior part of the tibia: (4) Solid fixation bone graft into bone bed by Kirschner wire or plate and screw and plaste cast: (5) The needed length of the Kirschner wire is calculated on the basis of the expected length of the leg after the affected bone and fibrous tissues have been removed and after the angular deformity has been corrected; (6) The Kirschner wire will be removed when solid clinical and radiographic union were apparent (mean more than two years); and (7) Prolonged orthotic protection was required when ankle transfixation had been performed and a knee-ankle-foot orthosis was worn until the patient reached skeletal maturity.

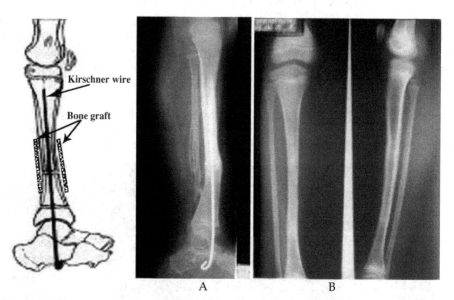

A   B

Fig. 17. A. PostOperative 6 months; B. Postoperative union of Pseudarthrosis 12 years 8 months (From Author - Hung NN. Use of an intramedullary Kirschner wire for treatment of congenital pseudarthrosis of the tibia in children. Journal of Pediatric Orthopaedics B 2009; 18:79–85 [21]).

8. Complications

Complications for grafts from the iliac crest

Some of the potential risks and complications of bone grafts employing the iliac crest as a donor site include:

8.1 Anterior Ilium

Pain

Pain after bone graft harvest from the anterior ilium has multiple origins. It can result from hematoma, wound infection, neuropraxia of cutaneous nerves, stress fracture, or from the dissection itself. Pain, from whatever the source, has been noted to last on average 3.75 weeks. In 90% of patients, symptoms resolve in less than 1 month but 2.8% may have persistent pain lasting over 3 months [29]

Cosmesis

Obtaining bone from the anterior ilium most often requires an additional incision from the recipient site incision. The overall cosmesis has been rated as good in 86.1%, fair in 10.4% and poor in 3.5%. Additionally, it has been observed that worse ratings are given by women and those who are obese [29]. Methods to improve cosmesis include using a trap door or subcrestal window technique to remove the graft allowing for preservation of the natural contour of the ilium [30]

Wound healing

Wound healing complications are not uncommon after bone graft harvest and have multiple origins, including infection, hematoma and wound dehiscence. Even with the use of thrombin-soaked gel foam and bone wax, residual bleeding often occurs from the cancellous bone. Studies have shown the presence of hematomas in 4-10% of patients [30]. Additionally, multiple vessels, including the deep circumflex, iliolumbar, and fourth lumbar arteries, may be damaged.

Nerve damage

Injury to the lateral femoral cutaneous and the ilioinguinal nerves is not an uncommon complication from anterior graft harvest. Meralgia paresthetica may occur when the lateral femoral cutaneous nerve is injured. There are three origins of injury to this nerve: neurotmesis of the nerve as it crosses the crest, neuropraxia from retraction of the iliacus and crush injury during stripping of the outer table muscles [30]. Symptoms include pain and numbness over the anterolateral thigh immediately postoperatively, and these symptoms are commonly worse with walking [31]. For this reason it is recommended to stop the skin incision and dissection 2 cm lateral to the ASIS.

Hernia

Herniation of abdominal contents through a bone graft site has been reported and can be a potentially serious complication requiring reoperation [30]. Abdominal wall muscles attach to the iliac crest and prevent abdominal contents from migrating over the crest, and the iliacus muscle prevents contents from penetrating through a defect in the iliac wing. The hernia forms when there has been a violation of these muscles with an inadequate repair [30]. It can be diagnosed clinically with confirmation by CT scan.

Pelvic fracture

The sartorius and tensor fascia lata originate on the ASIS and have been reported to cause an avulsion fracture to the ASIS. Hu and Bohlman [32] examined this and found that a graft taken 30mm posterior to the ASIS was 2.4 times the strength of a graft taken at 15mm. Therefore, it is recommended that any vertical cut into the ilium be at least 3 cm posterior to the ASIS [33]. Osteoporotic, elderly women have been found to be at a higher risk for this complication [34].

Gluteal gait

A gluteal gait is an abductor lurch seen as a result of abductor weakness, especially the gluteus medius. This may be found in up to 3% of patients after graft harvest [30]. Its incidence can be minimized through a less extensive stripping of the outer table muscles of the ilium and by careful reapproximation and secure reattachment of the gluteal fascia to the periosteum.

8.2 Posterior Ilium

Pain

Chronic pain, hyperesthesia and dysesthesia are among the most common complaints after posterior iliac bone graft harvest. Studies have shown that 29% of patients complain of chronic pain for longer than 1 year. It also has been shown that patients who have the bone graft taken for spinal reconstruction surgery have twice the incidence of pain compared with those who have the graft taken for spinal trauma purposes.

Hematoma or wound Infection

Hematomas have been found to be less problematic with posterior compared with anterior iliac graft harvests. This is thought to be secondary to the hemostatic effect of the body placing pressure on the surgical site.3,6 Although this may decrease hematoma formation, it has been observed that more than 10% of patients present with wound healing problems. Although the overall majority of complications are mild to moderate wound dehiscence, a 2.7% deep infection rate has been observed that required treatment with intravenous antibiotics [35].

Nerve injury

The nerves most commonly at risk are the superior cluneal nerves. Injury to the superior cluneal nerves may result in pain, hyperesthesia or paresthesia of the buttock region [30]. These nerves pierce the lumbodorsal fascia and cross the posterior iliac crest 6-8 cm lateral to the PSIS. They travel in the inferolateral direction [36, 37]. These nerves are intimately associated with the lumbodorsal fascia making their identification difficult. Previously it was believed that a vertical midline incision avoided the superior cluneal nerves and resulted in less postoperative pain than a lateral oblique incision. Fernyhough et al [36] failed to show a statistically significant difference in pain between the use of the lateral oblique incision and the vertical incision, thus concluding that either approach is appropriate.

Vascular injury

The superior gluteal artery exits the sciatic notch in the superior most portion and sends branches to the gluteal muscles. Careless placement of a retractor or removal of graft from the sciatic notch may result in laceration of the artery or arteriovenous fistula formation [30, 36]. In a cadaver study by Xu et al [37] the anatomic distances between the superior gluteal vessels and the pelvic landmarks were measured. The vessels were found to be an average of 62mm from the PSIS and 102mm from the iliac crest [37]. Injury can best be avoided by knowing the anatomy. The inferior margin of the roughened area just anterior and lateral to the PSIS should be the caudal limit for bone harvest, and should a retractor be used, it should not be blindly inserted into the sciatic notch. When vascular injury occurs, the artery may retract into the pelvis making visibility difficult.

Sacro-iliac (SI) joint instability

Cases of instability and dislocation of the SI joint have been reported after posterior iliac bone harvest. There are many ligaments that make up the SI joint complex. Most notably are the dense interosseous ligaments that are more numerous superiorly and offer the primary support. In addition, there are the short and long posterior ligaments and the thin anterior ligaments, which assist in the support. Compromise of these ligaments can result in instability and over time may result in pubic rami fractures and possible dislocation of the SI joint [38]

Ureteral injury

Ureteral injury is a very rare complication but important because of its severity. The ureters run deep through the sciatic notch and use of electrocautery or careless placement of a retractor can cause injury. Presenting symptoms may include fever, ileus, hematuria and hydronephrosi [30, 36].

8.3 Proximal tibial graft

Fracture

The most feared complication of tibial bone graft is the risk of fracture. O'Keeffe et al [39] reported one nondisplaced fracture of the tibial eminence. This was treated with nonweightbearing in a knee immobilizer and healed without further complication. Thor [40] and Van Damme and Merkx [41] reported fractures of the tibial metaphysis in the early postoperative period [42]. One was after a fall and required operative fixation. The other two were secondary to running and playing tennis, which led to the recommendation that impact activities and sports be avoided for 4-6 weeks postoperatively.

Removal of fibular graft

In the removal of a fibular graft three points should receive consideration: (1) the peroneal nerve must not be damaged; (2) the distal fourth of the bone must be left to maintain a stable ankle; and (3) the peroneal muscles should not be cut. (4) Nounion of fibula is removed.

Peroneal injury

If the transplant is to substitute for the distal end of the radius or for the distal end of the fibula, resect the proximal third of the fibula through the proximal end of the Henry approach and take care to avoid damaging the peroneal nerve. Expose the nerve first at the posteromedial aspect of the distal end of the biceps femoris tendon and trace it distally to where it winds around the neck of the fibula. In this location the nerve is covered by the origin of the peroneus longus muscle. Peroneal injury could be reduction of movement some anterolatral leg muscles.

Knee instability

With the back of the knife blade toward the nerve, divide the thin slip of peroneus longus muscle bridging it. Then displace the nerve from its normal bed into an anterior position. As the dissection continues, protect the anterior tibial vessels that pass between the neck of the fibula and the tibia by subperiosteal dissection. After the resection is complete, must to suture the biceps tendon and the fibular collateral ligament to the adjacent soft tissues to create knee stability.

Ankle instability

If the distal fourth of the bone is removed, must be left to maintain a stable ankle by apply a cast from below the knee to the base of the toes or distal tibia-fibula fixation by screw. The cast or screw were removed when solid clinical and radiographic fibular union was apparent

Muscular weakness after removal of a portion of the fibula

The entire proximal two thirds of the fibula may be removed without materially disabling the leg. However, a study by Gore et al [43] indicates that most patients have complaints and mild muscular weakness after removal of a portion of the fibula. The configuration of the proximal end of the fibula is an advantage: the proximal end has a rounded prominence, which is partially covered by hyaline cartilage, and thus forms a satisfactory transplant to replace the distal third of the radius or the distal third of the fibula. After transplantation the hyaline cartilage probably degenerates rapidly into a fibrocartilaginous surface; even so, this surface is preferable to raw bone.

9. Complications of allograft

Nonunion

Nonunion, by convention, implies nonhealing of the graft–host junction at 1 year and has been reported from 11 to 30% [44 - 47]. Factors that have been implicated are age (older age), type of graft (highest in arthrodesis), location (worse for diaphyseal junction), stage of disease (higher for stage 2 or 3), requirement of adjuvant therapy (higher for chemotherapy or radiotherapy), infection, fracture, type and stability of fixation, and revision surgery (worse as number of procedures increase) [44, 47, 48]. Infection and fracture rates are higher in patients with nonunions and subsequent outcomes are poorer. Apart from these mechanical reasons, immunological response may also play a part in nonunion [44, 49]. To treat nonunions, various procedures have been recommended, including autogenous bone graft, double plating for stable fixation, and vascularized fibular grafts [44].

Fractures

Allograft fracture has been seen in 12–54% of cases, depending on the variables involved and the definition of fracture [49 - 55]. Fractures generally occur after 6 months, around the time of revascularization; most fractures (75%) occur during the first 3 years of implantation [51]. Chemotherapy, radiation, cortical penetrating internal fixation, nonunion at host–graft junction, infection, type of graft (higher for osteoarticular and arthrodesis transplant), location (more for femur), gap more than 2 mm, and larger grafts (more than 14.5 cm) have been linked with fracture in various studies [15, 47, 51, 53 - 58].

Infection

Infection is the most devastating complication after allograft transplant, often the leading cause of graft failure. It is associated with other complications and a worse outcome. The incidence has been reported to be 9–30% [45, 59 - 64]. About 75% were diagnosed within the first 4 months after implantation in the study by Lord et al. [62] and 70% within the first month in a study by Dick and Strauch [61]. Polymicrobial infection may be present in 50% of the cases and Staphylococcus epidermidis may be the most common single organism [61, 63]. Factors associated with local wound problems are an extensive surgery (tumor stage, more bone, soft tissue or skin loss, duration of surgery, postoperative hematoma or drainage), adjuvant therapy, the patient's immune status and multiple surgeries [61, 63]. Late infection is unrelated to adjuvant therapy and may happen anytime [65].

Graft disease transmission

Donor screening is the first step in preventing the use of contaminated grafts [66]. Both the FDA and AATB have detailed guidelines regarding the medical history as well as clinical test results of the donor. Screening is currently done for HIV, hepatitis B virus, hepatitis C virus, human transmissible spongiform encephalopathy, syphilis, human T-lymphotropic virus, and cytomegalovirus. Bone allograft contamination is rare, and in a previous study had been estimated to be less than 0.3% [67]. The number of actual infections from allografts is very low: two reports of HIV in 1988, 1992; three reports of hepatitis, hepatitis B in 1954, hepatitis C in 1992, 1993. and one fatal clostridium transmission in 1995 [68]. When examining graft tissue, however, one study reported five (18.5%) of 27 femoral heads from live donors and three (37.5%) of eight allografts from cadavers to be infected [69].

10. Conclusion

Autogenous bone graft continues to be the gold standard for the filling of bone defects in spinal surgery, trauma and treatment of malunions, nonunions and tumors. Each site of autologous bone graft has its advantages and disadvantages, including the anatomic location, which may make one site preferable over another, depending on the graft recipient site. With the increasing use of bone substitutes, it is important to understand all the risks of autogenous bone harvest before possibly exposing a patient to one of the rare but potentially serious complications.

In 2005, over 0.8 million bone and tissue allografts were distributed in the United States [70]. All orthopedic surgeons should understand not only the biologic properties of grafts, but also the methods and regulation of tissue collection. In 85% of the 340 surveyed institutions, grafts were selected by nonorthopedic personnel [45]. It is incumbent on the surgeon tomake an informed decision in order to achieve the best outcome each time an allograft is used.

11. Acknowledgements

I would like to thank assistance of our two research assistants in the Orthopaedic Department at National Hospital for Paediatrics, Dr. Le Tuan Anh and Dr. Hoang Hai Duc are greatly appreciated in general assistance in manuscript preparation.

In particular, I thank Dr. Tran Phan Ninh and Dr. Do Thanh Tung in the Diagnostic Imaging Department at National Hospital for Paediatrics for the enormous effort they put in to locate suitable illustrations for the book by sifting through thousands of images.

I am grateful to my wife, Do Ngoc Yen, and my daughters, HienTan and HongCuong, for tolerating my absences to the study to put those ramblings onto the computer.

12. Dedication

To my dearest wife, Do Ngoc Yen, and my daughters, HienTan and HongCuong, who have accepted, with great tolerance and understanding, the lack of a husband and father due to firstly the demands of a medical career and secondly to help prepare this text.

13. References

[1] Harkins HN, Phemister DB. Simplified Technic of Onlay Grafts. JAMA. 1937;109:1501

[2] Phemister DB. The Fate of Transplanted Bone and Re generative Power of Its Various Constituents. Surg Gynecol Obstet 1914;19:303

[3] Abbott LC, Schottstaedt ER, Saunders JB, et al. The Evaluation of Cortical and Cancellous Bone as Grafting Material. A Clinical and Experimental Study. J Bone Joint Surg. 1947; 29:381 - 414

[4] Ray RD, Sabet TY. Bone Grafts: Cellular Survival Versus Induction. J Bone Joint Surg. 1963;45-A: 337 - 344

[5] Arora BK, Laskin DM. Sex Chromatin as a Cellular Label of Osteogenesis by Bone Grafts. J Bone Joint Surg. 1964; 46-A: 1269 - 1276

[6] Ray RD. Vascularization of Bone Grafts and Implants. Clin Orthop. 1972; 87: 43 - 51

[7] Chase SW, Herndon CH. The Fate of Autogenous and Homogenous Bone Grafts: A Historical Review. J Bone Joint Surg. 1955; 37-A: 809 - 841

[8] Delloye C, Verhelpen M, d' Hemricourt J, et al. Morphometric and Physical Investigations of Segmental Cortical Bone Autografts in Canine Ulnar Defects. Clin Orthop. 1992; 282: 273 - 885

[9] Enneking WF, Morris JL. Human Autologous Cortical Bone Transplants. Clin Orthop. 1972; 87: 28 - 39

[10] Enneking WF, Burchardt H, Puhl J, et al. Physical and Biologic Aspects of Repair in Dog Cortical Bone Transplants. J Bone Joint Surg. 1975; 57-A: 237 - 252

[11] Burchardt H, Glowczewskie FP, Enneking WF. Allogenic Segmental Fibular Transplants in Azathioprine-immunosuppressed Dogs. J Bone Joint Surg. 1977; 59-A: 881-894.

[12] Brien RE, Terek RM, Healey JH, Lane JM. Allograft Reconstruction after Proximal Tibial Resection for Bone Tumors. Clin Orthop. 1994; 303: 116 - 128

[13] Buttermann GR, Glazer PA, Bradford DS. The Use of Bone Allografts in the Spine. Clin Orthop. 1996; 324: 75 - 89

[14] Gross AE, Silverstein EA, Fal J, et al. The Allotransplantation of Partial Joints in the Treatment of Osteoarthritis of the Knee. Clin Orthop. 1975;108:7 - 21

[15] Ottolenghi CE. Massive Osteocarticular Bone Grafts. Technique and Results of 62 Cases. Clin Orthop. 1972; 87: 156 - 170

[16] Albee FH. Transplantation of a Portion of the Tibia into the Spine for Pott's Disease. JAMA. 1911; 57: 85 - 98

[17] Albee FH. Evolution of Bone Graft Surgery. Am J Surg. 1944; 63: 421 - 536

[18] Aurori BF, Weierman RJ, Lowell HA, et al. Pseudarthrosis after Spinal Fusion for Scoliosis. Clin Orthop. 1985; 199: 153 - 167

[19] Bassett CAL. Clinical Implications of Cell Function in Bone Grafting. Clin Orthop. 1972; 87: 49 - 63

[20] Boyd HB, Lapinski SP. Causes and Treatment of Non union of the Shafts of the Long Bones. In American Academy of Orthopaedic Surgeons: Instructional Course Lectures, Vol. 17. St. Louis: C.V. Mosby; 1960

[21] Hung NN. Use of an intramedullary Kirschner wire for treatment of congenital pseudarthrosis of the tibia in children. Journal of Pediatric Orthopaedics B. 2009; 18: 79–85

[22] Albee FH. Transplantation of a Portion of the Tibia into the Spine for Pott's Disease. JAMA. 1911; 57: 85 - 108

[23] Albee FH. Evolution of Bone Graft Surgery. Am J Surg. 1944; 63:421 - 436

[24] Shapiro MS, Endrizzi DP, Cannon RM, Dick HM. Treatment of Tibial Defects and Nonunions Using ipsilateral Vascularized Fibular Transposition. Clin Orthop. 1993;296:207 - 223

[25] Meyers MH, Harvey JP, Moore TM. Treatment of Displaced Subcapital and Transcervical Fractures of the Femoral Neck by Muscle-Pedicle Bone Graft and Internal Fixation. J Bone Joint Surg. 1973; 55-A:257 - 274

[26] Meyers MH, Harvey JP, Moore TM. The Muscle-Pedicle Bone Graft in the Treatment of Displaced Fractures of the Femoral Neck: Indications, Operative Technique, and Results. Orthop Clin North Am. 1974;5:779 - 794

[27] McMaster PE, Hohl M. Tibiofibular Cross-peg Grafting. J Bone Joint Surg. 1965; 47-A:1146 - 1158.

[28] Langenskiöld A: Pseudarthrosis of the Fibula and Progressive Valgus Deformity of the Ankle in Children: Treatment by Fusion of the Distal Tibial and Fibular Metaphyses REVIEW OF THREE CASES. The Journal Bone and Joint Surg. 1967 ; 49-A (3): 463-470

[29] Schnee CL, Freese A, Weil RJ, Marcotte PJ. Analysis of harvest morbidity and radiographic outcome using autograft for anterior cervical fusion. Spine. 1997; 22: 2222- 2227

[30] Kurz LT, Garfin SR, Booth RE. Harvesting autogenous iliac bone grafts: a review of complications and techniques. Spine. 1989; 14:1324-1331.

[31] Weikel AM, Habal MB. Meralgia paresthetica: a complication of iliac bone procurement. Plast Reconstr Surg. 1977; 60:572-574

[32] Hu RW, Bohlman HH. Fracture at the iliac bone graft harvest site after fusion of the spine. Clin Orthop Relat Res. 1994; 309: 208-213.

[33] Ebraheim NA, Yang H, Lu J, Biyani A. Anterior iliac crest bone graft: anatomic considerations. Spine. 1997; 22: 847-849

[34] Alt V, Nawab A, Seligson D. Bone grafting from the proximal tibia. Trauma. 1999; 47:555-557.

[35] Sasso RC, Williams JI, Dimasi N, Meyer PR . Postoperative drains at the donor sites of iliac-crest bone grafts. J Bone Joint Surg. 1998; 80-A: 631-635.

[36] Fernyhough JC, Schimandle JJ, Weigel MC, Edwards CC, Levine AM . Chronic donor site pain complication bone graft harvesting from the posterior iliac crest for spinal fusion. Spine. 1992; 17:1474-1480.

[37] Xu R, Haman SP, Ebraheim NA, Yeasting RA:. Anatomic considerations for posterior iliac bone harvesting. Spine. 1996; 21:1017-1020.

[38] Lichtblau S. Dislocation of the sacro-iliac joint: a complication of bone grafting. J Bone Joint Surg. 1962; 44-A:193-198

[39] O'Keeffe RM, Riemer BL, Butterfield SL. Harvesting of autogenous cancellous bone graft from the proximal tibial metaphysis: a review of 230 cases. J Orthop Trauma. 1991; 5: 469-474

[40] Thor A, Farzad P, Larsson S. Fracture of the tibia: complication of bone grafting to the anterior maxilla. Brit J Oral Maxillofac Surg. 2006; 44: 46-48.

[41] Van Damme PA, Merkx MA. A modification of tibial bone-graft harvesting technique. Int J Oral Maxillofac Surg. 1996; 25: 346-348.

[42] Younger EM, Chapman MW. Morbidity at bone graft donor sites. J Orthop Trauma. 1989; 3:192-195.

[43] Gore DR, Brechbuler M. Treatment of nonunions following anterior cervical discectomy and fusion with interspinous wiring and bone grafting. J Surg Orthop.2003;12(4): 214-221.

[44] Hornicek FJ, Gebhardt MC, Tomford WW, et al. Factors affecting nonunion of the allograft-host junction. Clin Orthop Relat Res. 2001; 382: 87–98.

[45] Mankin HJ, Gebhardt MC, Jennings LC, et al. Long-term results of allograft replacement in the management of bone tumors. Clin Orthop Relat Res. 1996; 324:86–97.

[46] Ortiz-Cruz E, Gebhardt MC, Jennings LC, et al. The results of transplantation of intercalary allografts after resection of tumors. A long-term follow-up study. J Bone Joint Surg Am. 1997; 79A: 97–106.

[47] Vander Griend RA. The effect of internal fixation on the healing of large allografts. J Bone Joint Surg Am. 1994; 76A:657–663.

[48] Muscolo DL, Ayerza MA, Aponte-Tinao L, et al. Intercalary femur and tibia segmental allografts provide an acceptable alternative in reconstructing tumor resections. Clin Orthop Relat Res. 2004; 426:97–102.

[49] Malinin TI, Buck BE, Temple HT, et al. Incidence of clostridial contamination in donors' musculoskeletal tissue. J Bone Joint Surg Br. 2003; 85B:1051–1054.

[50] Alman BA, De Bari A, Krajbich JI. Massive allografts in the treatment of osteosarcoma and Ewing sarcoma in children and adolescents. J Bone Joint Surg Am, 1995; 77A:54–64

[51] Berrey BH Jr, Lord CF, Gebhardt MC, Mankin HJ. Fractures of allografts. Frequency, treatment, and end-results. J Bone Joint Surg Am. 1990; 72A:825–833.

[52] San-Julian M, Canadell J. Fractures of allografts used in limb preserving operations. Int Orthop. 1998; 22:32–36.

[53] Sorger JI, Hornicek FJ, Zavatta M, et al. Allograft fractures revisited. Clin Orthop Relat Res. 2001; 382:66–74

[54] Thompson RC Jr, Garg A, Clohisy DR, Cheng EY. Fractures in large-segment allografts. Clin Orthop Relat Res. 2000; 370: 227–235.

[55] San-Julian M, Canadell J. Fractures of allografts used in limb preserving operations. Int Orthop. 1998; 22:32–36.

[56] Thompson RC Jr, Pickvance EA, Garry D. Fractures in large-segment allografts. J Bone Joint Surg Am. 1993; 75A: 1663–1673

[57] Deijkers RL, Bloem RM, Kroon HM, et al. Epidiaphyseal versus other intercalary allografts for tumors of the lower limb. Clin Orthop Relat Res. 2005; 439:151–160.

[58] Lietman SA, Tomford WW, Gebhardt MC, et al. Complications of irradiated allografts in orthopaedic tumor surgery. Clin Orthop Relat Res. 2000; 375: 214–217

[59] Donati D, Capanna R, Campanacci D, et al. The use of massive bone allografts for intercalary reconstruction and arthrodeses after tumor resection. A multicentric European study. Chir Organi Mov. 1993; 78: 81–94.

[60] Donati D, Di Liddo M, Zavatta M, et al. Massive bone allograft reconstruction in high-grade osteosarcoma. Clin Orthop Relat Res. 2000; 377: 186–194.

[61] Dick HM, Strauch RJ. Infection of massive bone allografts. Clin Orthop Relat Res. 1994; 306:46–53.

[62] Gebhardt MC, Flugstad DI, Springfield DS, Mankin HJ. The use of bone allografts for limb salvage in high-grade extremity osteosarcoma. Clin Orthop Relat Res. 1991; 270:181–196

[63] Lord CF, Gebhardt MC, Tomford WW,Mankin HJ. Infection in bone allografts. Incidence, nature, and treatment. J Bone Joint Surg Am. 1988; 70A:369–376.

[64] Mankin HJ, Friedlaender GE, Tomford WW. Massive allograft transplantation following tumor resection. In: Friedlaender GE, Mankin HJ, Goldberg VM, editors. Bone grafts and bone graft substitutes; 2006. Rosemont: American Academy of Orthopaedic Surgeons; pp. 39–47

[65] Matejovsky Z Jr, Matejovsky Z, Kofranek I. Massive allografts in tumour surgery. Int Orthop. 2006; 30: 478–483.

[66] Eastlund T. Bacterial infection transmitted by human tissue allograft transplantation. Cell Tissue Bank. 2006; 7: 147–166.

[67] Tomford WW, Starkweather RJ, Goldman MH. A study of the clinical incidence of nfection in the use of banked allograft bone. J Bone Joint Surg Am. 1981; 63A: 244–248

[68] Tomford WW. Transmission of disease through transplantation of musculoskeletal allografts. J Bone Joint Surg Am. 1995; 77A:1742–1754.

[69] Chapman PG, Villar RN. The bacteriology of bone allografts. J Bone Joint Surg Br. 1992; 74B: 398–399.

[70] Delloye C, Cornu O, Druez V, Barbier O. Bone allografts. What they can offer and what they cannot. J Bone Joint Surg Br. 2007; 89B: 574–579.

[71] Lavernia CJ, Malinin TI, Temple HT, Moreyra CE. Bone and tissue allograft use by orthopaedic surgeons. J Arthroplasty. 2004; 19: 430–435.

Part 2

Basic Science

3

Influence of Freeze-Drying and Irradiation on Mechanical Properties of Human Cancellous Bone: Application to Impaction Bone Grafting

Olivier Cornu

Orthopaedic and Trauma Department, Cliniques Universitaires St-Luc,
Université Catholique de Louvain, Brussels,
Belgium

1. Introduction

The use of a solid bone graft to restore bone stock and insure implant stability in hip revision surgery was introduced by Harris et al. (1). Better results have been obtained on the femoral site than on the acetabulum where high failure rate has been reported at ten years (2-7). Progressively, a new technique for restoring the acetabulum emerged with the concept of bone impaction which was introduced by Slooff et al. and later extended to the femur by Ling et al. (8-9). The technique consists in impacting bone chips with a phantom into the contained femoral or acetabular defect to produce a layer of tightly impacted bone where an implant shall be inserted with the cement being pressurized into the graft during cementation. Clinical results of impaction bone grafting techniques were largely improved with re-revision rates comparable to those observed after primary arthroplasty (10-12). Acetabular reconstructions were described as requiring between one and three femoral heads (12) and femoral impactions two or more, based on the preoperative bone loss (13-14).

As bone impaction became a recognised modality for bone reconstruction, the demand for bone allograft sharply increased. Consequently, an existing shortfall in the supply of banked bone was predicted to increase (15-16). As the impaction technique had been set up with frozen material, most bone banks were facing difficulties to provide frozen femoral heads (17). The increase in the number of hip arthroplasties did not mirror a concurrent increase in banked femoral heads. Indeed, the rate of rejection remained high (16) whereas the formal 6-month visit to get out the quarantine was difficult to obtained.

Concerns were raised about the possibility of an occult pathology into a femoral head, which could not have been identified through careful history and when different authors reported an incidence of 5 to 8% (18-19). Bacterial contamination rate reported with cadaver bone harvesting was another concern that limited supply from another source of fresh frozen bone (20).

Bone processing which allows a complete removal of bone marrow and cell debris from the bone and the machining of the material represented a potential solution to overcome these problems. However, no study had been reported comparing the mechanical stability of a femur and acetabulum restored with either impacted frozen bone morsels or freeze-dried ones. The bone marrow content was considered to be important for the graft stickiness which influenced the biological and mechanical properties in impaction bone grafting (21). Although each separate step of the bone process did not appear to influence the bone strength (22-27), surgeons reported that freeze-dried bone was brittle and hence, unsuitable for being fixed and trimmed during surgery (28). However, the cumulative effects of every applied treatment were known to impact the mechanical properties of the musculo-skeletal tissue (29-30).

This chapter will cover the influences of various parameters (bone processing, freeze-drying, irradiation, processing sequence and temperature during irradiation) on the mechanical properties of cancellous bone. Mechanical damage due to irradiation will be related to damage of the collagen protein. Benefits of defatting, freeze-drying and irradiation in terms of osteoconductivity and tissue safety will be further discussed.

Application of processed freeze-dried irradiated bone to impaction bone grafting technique will be considered. The embrittlement theory and the influence of particle sizes will be presented to explain how processed bone is suitable to meet the mechanical demand of hip revision surgery. Results will be discussed and compared in more realistic surgical situations by observing implant stability after frozen or freeze-dried irradiated bone impaction. Finally, bone graft remodelling will be discussed.

2. Influence of various parameters on cancellous bone: Bone processing, freeze-drying, irradiation, processing sequence and temperature during irradiation

2.1 Mechanical effects of drying, freeze-drying and defatting

The effect of drying and rewetting on the mechanical properties of cortical bone was thought to be negligible because changes of the mechanical properties were very limited and considered as insignificant (31). Prolonged storage of bone in frozen state or in ethanol solution did not change the bone stiffness of trabecular bone, and neither did several thawing and refreezing sequences (32). Defatting combined with dehydration made the bone stiffer and brittle (32). The importance of re-hydration of a bone that has been dried was further emphasized by Conrad et al., as non rehydrated dried bones appeared to be both stronger and stiffer than their rehydrated counterparts (33). After 24 hours rehydration, freeze-dried grafts compared with frozen grafts showed no significant difference in mean compressive strength. An average gain of 40 % of the compressive strength and stiffness was recovered after one-hour rehydration in vacuo. The same observation was done by Bright and Burchardt on cortical bone (23). Complete restorations of the mechanical parameters after rehydration were also reported by Pelker et al. and Thoren et al. (24, 27). These authors did not find a significant difference in the compressive strength of freeze-dried rehydrated bone compared with normal bone in a rat vertebral model (24) and did not observe difference in the biomechanical properties of rehydrated bone after lipid extraction with chloroform methanol (27).

In our experiments, defatting and freeze-drying caused just a slight reduction in the ultimate compressive strength and stiffness but did not affect the work to failure, due to a higher ductility (34). In contrast to the observations of Bright and Burstein and Conrad et al.

works (33, 35) who noted that 24h were required for regaining the natural mechanical properties of the bone, a short 30-minute period of rehydration was enough to make bone more resilient.

Slight influence of physical or chemical defatting of cancellous bone grafts was recently confirmed (36-37). Other authors investigated biomechanical properties of the cortical and trabecular bone after high pressure lavage. Young's modulus and ultimate strength did not decrease after exposure to 300 MPa. After pressure treatment at 600 MPa, Young's modulus and ultimate strength respectively remained almost unchanged in trabecular bone and were reduced about 15% in cortical bone (38).

2.2 Mechanical effects of irradiation and sequences of freeze-drying and irradiation

2.2.1 Irradiation of a frozen bone

Gamma irradiation at a dose of 25 kGy has no apparent detrimental effect on cancellous bone strength. The mean values obtained in our experiments were within the range of values commonly observed for human bone that has been exposed to as high as 50 kGy (39). Anderson et al. reported earlier a 60% reduction of compressive strength and modulus for doses at or above 60 kGy (40). Their data were in agreement with our observations that processed frozen irradiated bone under dry ice did not show any detrimental effect after a 30 kGy irradiation.

2.2.2 Irradiation at room temperature of a freeze-dried bone

However at a 25 kGy dose at room temperature, alteration in the mechanical properties of cortical bone in compression occurred in the plastic modulus whereas the elastic domain remained unchanged. The capacity to absorb work before failure was also decreased in a dose-dependent manner (41-42). Similarly torque resistance of the frozen bone was greatly impaired with gamma-irradiation at a dose of 25kGy (43).

Our data for freeze-dried irradiated at room temperature cancellous bone are similar to the observation from Currey et al. and Hamer et al. (34, 41-42). The quantification of the post yield parameters showed that irradiation of freeze-dried cancellous bone at 25 kGy and at room temperature mainly reduced the capacity for energy absorption by shrinking the post-yield strain. Whether bone brittleness was due to irradiation on freeze-dried bone alone or temperature during irradiation or to a synergetic effect of the freeze-drying-irradiation process could not be yet assessed. Therefore, an inverted sequence of the freeze-drying-irradiation process and irradiation under dry ice was also examined.

2.2.3 Sequence of order and irradiation under dry ice

Performing freeze-drying either before or after irradiation under dry ice decreased the ultimate stress from 30% and the work to failure from 40% and impaired the results obtained with irradiation or freeze-drying separately. Stiffness was more preserved when freeze-drying preceded irradiation. The plastic domain of the strain-stress curve was more adversely affected by the usual freeze-drying-irradiation at room temperature sequence. Performing freeze-drying after irradiation allowed strain preservation but work to failure was decreased due to the stiffness and stress drops (Figure 1).

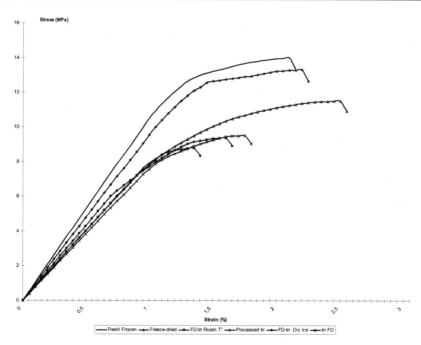

Compressive mechanical properties of cancellous bone are not influenced by irradiation under dry ice and supported moderate changes with freeze-drying. Negative synergetic effects of combined freeze-drying-irradiation processes are observed whatever the temperature during irradiation cycle. Irradiation cycle was performed within 3h00 at a 25 kGy dose rate. The curves were drawn proportionally to the observed mean values.

Fig. 1. Comparison of typical stress-strain curves. Strain-stress curves observed after freeze-drying, irradiation and sequence of both at two different temperatures.

Negative cumulative effect of freeze-drying and irradiation was already noted by Bright et al. and Triantafyllou et al. on cortical bone (25, 44). Preserving freeze-dried graft under dry ice during irradiation limited the damage compare to the same sequence at room temperature. These observations were consistent with the report of Hamer et al. (45), who found that cortical bone irradiated at –78°C was less brittle and had less collagen damage than when irradiated at room temperature.

2.3 Irradiation and collagen

Bright and Burchardt considered that a bone that has been freeze-dried and irradiated resembled to bone from old patient in term of mechanics. They thought that alterations were due to changes in the bone collagen cross-linking (23). Significant decrease in hydroxypyridinium cross-link density was reported after irradiation of bone tendon bone patellar allograft with significant correlation of dose dependant reduction of modulus properties (46). It was further suggested that gamma radiation might have less effect on the collagen structure in older bone because there were fewer reductible cross-links than in younger one (47).

Adding glucose, which in theory can initiate cross-link formation in collagen during exposure to gamma-irradiation, allowed collagen films containing glucose to have significantly greater mechanical properties and resistance to enzymatic degradation compared with controls. Nevertheless, gel electrophoresis showed that glucose did not prevent peptide fragmentation and therefore, the higher strength and stability in glucose-incorporated collagen films might be due to glucose-derived cross-links (48). Thiourea has been selected as a free radical scavenger and demonstrated a positive effect on the fracture energy of thiourea treated-irradiated bones than those of the irradiated bones. Irradiated specimens did not exhibit a noteworthy amount of intact alpha-chains whereas those irradiated in the presence of thiourea demonstrated intact alpha-chains. The damage occurred through the cleavage of the collagen backbone (49).

Drózdz et al. found a significant decrease in total collagen content resulting from the reduction of salt-soluble and acid-soluble collagen fractions (50). He estimated that an increased content of insoluble collagen fraction may confirm the opinion about stimulative gamma-rays influence upon cross-links formation. His observations were confirmed by Nguyen et al. who reported that irradiation caused release of free radicals resulting from radiolysis of water molecules and inducing cross-linking reactions in collagen molecules in wet specimens and split polypeptide chains (51). This hypothesis of the damaged first-order structure of the collagen macromolecule was also supported by Marzec et al. (52).

Differences in the mechanical behaviour after the different freeze-drying-irradiation-temperature sequences may be explained by the variation in active oxygen free radicals formation due to ionizing radiation. Free radicals are obtained by water radiolyis and their ability to move and interact with the material may be impaired when this one is frozen (53). The increased damages observed in absence of free water in pre-dried specimen may be due to direct damages to the proteins by irradiation, suggesting a higher sensitivity of freeze-dried proteins to irradiation than hydrated ones. This is supported by the observation of better osteoinductive properties of demineralised powder when irradiated in the hydrated frozen state (54). Collagen degradation by irradiation may account for the accelerate graft remodelling (54-55).

The good compressive mechanical performance of processed frozen irradiated cancellous bone shall be considered cautiously in regard with potential collagen damage. The impairment of the mechanical function of gamma radiation sterilized cortical allografts is even worse in fatigue and may increase the risk of fracture (47, 49, 56).

2.4 Osteoconductivity of defatted bone

Extraction of lipids from cancellous bone before implantation increased the ingrowth of cells from the host enhancing the osteoconductivity of the bone (57). In this situation, the graft provided the template to guide the repairing tissue. Along with the increased new bone formation, there was a concomitant decrease of the grafted bone that led to a net increase of new bone when bone was defatted before implantation (27). This means that the grafted bone is progressively removed as a result of osteoclastic action and new bone from the host is deposited into the graft. This process of bone removal and new bone deposited has been called creeping-substitution. The amount of unresorbed graft remnant was higher in the unprocessed bone grafts than in the washed ones whether or not subsequently irradiated (58). This observation is consistent with an accelerate bone remodelling after irradiation.

Another argument for defatting the bone before implantation is that the removal of fat will avoid the peroxidation of lipids during radiation sterilisation as reported by Moreau et al (59). They further demonstrated that peroxidated lipids had a cytotoxic effect on cultured cells. Peroxidation of marrow fat was further incriminated in increasing apoptosis of osteoblasts and decreasing activity of osteoclasts when they were cultured onto irradiated bone slices (51). Finally, when processing was not performed in an aseptic manner, bacterial by-products can persist after irradiation and induce inflammatory bone resorption following macrophage activation (51).

2.5 Tissue safety: Freeze-drying, irradiation and processing

2.5.1 Freeze-drying

Lyophilisation of tissues is usually performed without cryoprotective agent and consequently there is no cell survival in a freeze-dried tissue. The finding that only recipients of frozen bone from an infected seronegative donor contracted human immunodeficiency virus has led to speculation that freeze-drying may render a retroviral-infected tissue non infectious. However, it has been demonstrated in a feline-leukemia-virus infected allograft model that freeze-drying did not inactivate retrovirus (60).

2.5.2 Irradiation

While Campbell et al. firstly reported retrovirus inactivation with a standard 25 kGy dose in a HTLV-IIIB virus infected cortical allograft model (61), he pointed out that the virus was a relatively radio-resistant organism, a property common to most viruses. This irradiation resistance was recognized by many authors who estimated that irradiation at 25 kGy did not appear to be effective enough for HIV virus (62-64). Campbell et al. noted that an irradiation dose required to inactivate the HIV bioburden in allograft bone should be 35 kGy and the irradiation dose required to achieve a sterility assurance level of 10^{-6} was 89 kGy (65). If irradiation is applied to a frozen hydrated specimen, it may be beneficial from a mechanical and biological point of view, but sterilizing effect may be lowered. It has been shown that HIV inactivation was decreased when irradiation was performed at low temperature on frozen plasma (66).

The radiosensitivity of hepatitis viruses is higher and clinical data suggest that hepatitis C-contaminated tissues did not transmit the virus after irradiation (67, 68). While high inactivation rate have been achieved with 50 kGy doses in virus infected bone allografts model (69, 70), it is actually concluded that gamma irradiation should be disregarded as a significant isolated virus inactivation method for bone allografts.

Prions are strongly resistant to radiation (71- 72) and therefore irradiation is unable to inactivate this pathogenic agent.

A standard 25 kGy irradiation is appropriate for bacterial sterilisation when a bio-burden control or a process validation have been performed. We have reported 7 to 9 logarithms bacterial reductions after 25 kGy irradiation of highly contaminated cancellous bone blocks (73). Analysis of Clostridium sordellii inactivation kinetics indicated that a 16 log10 reduction was obtained after 50 kGy (70). Contamination during bone preparation shall be strongly limited to allow sterility assurance level.

2.5.3 Processing

Processes based on multiple steps of inactivating treatments offer a cumulative effect and a striking reduction of the risk of disease transmission. Steps may be chosen on their ability to specifically inactivate pathogenic agents. Pulse lavage decontaminates tissue from bacterial microorganisms with one decimal reduction (74-75), while virus elimination was also reported after mechanical lavage of bone (76). Demineralization process inactivated infectious retrovirus in infected cortical bone, thereby preventing disease transmission (76-77).

Detergents are able to remote or inactivate coated viruses (78), while sodium hydroxide and sodium hypochlorite are effective against transmissible spongiform encephalopathy agent (79). Hydrogen peroxide produces free radicals and is effective against viruses and bacteria. Hydrogen peroxide and prion inactivating steps adopted in our bank (two steps out of twelve) have been validated with five representative or inactivating-agent-resistant viruses in a cancellous bone blocks model. Cumulative seven logarithm reductions have been obtained for all tested viruses. Similar viral inactivation rates were obtained with a multiple step process by Fages et al. (80).

No bacterial growth were observed after each step of the chemical process developed by our bank, while largely contaminated bone blocks with pathogenic, sporulated and environment resistant microorganisms were processed (73).

3. Mechanical consideration in impaction bone grafting

3.1 Changes in stiffness and compactness during impaction

3.1.1 Embrittlement theory

Freeze-drying and irradiation at room temperature make cancellous bone brittle. How can a softer material give a stiffer reconstruction? In our experiments, freeze-dried irradiated bone appeared to get impacted faster than the frozen control whatever the particle size (81-83). During an impaction bone grafting procedure, the stress is applied at such high speed that the flow of liquids may play an important role (84) and the replacement of bone marrow by saline in the processed bone may accelerate the grafts compaction (85). The faster reduction in height observed in our second experiments with the processed allografts series (defatted, defatted and freeze-dried, defatted and freeze-dried irradiated) might account for a rapid expulsion of liquid but stiffness and bone density increased faster and to a higher value in the irradiated group (82). The embrittlement due to the freeze-drying-irradiation sequence might enhance the compaction rate while the higher ductility of the freeze-dried but non irradiated bone reduced brittleness and might account for the lower compaction, stiffness and density obtained with this material.

Freeze-dried irradiated large particles were stiffer after 30 impactions than any other morsels. Nevertheless, these series showed a reduction of their stiffness for higher impaction rate and tended to the same stiffness as freeze dried small particles. Under significant loading, these trabeculae might fail with a fracture that loosened the particle interlock. Such loosening explains the stiffness reduction of the large freeze-dried and irradiated particles. This was supported by the loss of height and the final density of these series which are comparable to those from small freeze-dried particles. Structurally damaged cancellous bone is known to have a much lower elastic modulus (86). The preservation of the plastic mechanical properties as well as the presence of bone marrow in the frozen series may encounter of the lower compactness (85, 87-89) and the absence of collapsing in our models. The theory of bone embrittlement was further supported as compaction was faster when the grafts were morselised twice.

The mechanical properties of cancellous bone have been shown to be related to its apparent density, which depends on the porosity (90). Impacting freeze-dried irradiated bone created a layer that had a higher density and therefore a higher modulus, throughout the relationship between density and material properties cannot be fully applied to morselised bone, as the graft no longer has structural continuity (91).

3.1.2 Particle size influence

Particles sizing may also influence mechanical strength. For optimum shear strength, particles aggregate requires a mix of sizes represented by a logarithmic curve (92). While, none of the bone mills will produce an ideal profile, the particle size profile is larger when bigger particles are produced. In the clinical setting, an increase in the range size of particles has been obtained by putting bone through two different sizes of graters or passing some of the large graft morsels through the same mill twice.

3.1.2.1 The interlocking effect

Experimentally, we noted that preparation of well graded graft through a 1 mm beater mill (Retsch Cross beater mill SK100, Retsch GmbH, Haan, Germany) produced grafting material that was almost fluid. In our femoral model, these frozen particles did perform differently from those obtained with a rongeur, but not from those obtained with the Noviomagus bone mill. In the acetabular model, the particles were mechanically inferior in compaction and shear. These millimetric particles obtained from the Retsch mill was comparable to a fine powder, and filled a lower volume when placed in the impactor and showed higher density after few impactions but stiffness did not increase comparatively and remained lower than those from centimetric large particles. As suggested by authors, fresh frozen large particles got a higher stiffness than smaller morsels during impaction (92-95). This was due to the small size of the bone chips that did not allow an interlocking effect (96). The internal porosity of each morsel allowed deformation and causes them to interlock with each other during impaction (93).

This was coherent with our observation of an improved shear resistance of large particles. In our hands, acetabular reconstruction with ring reinforcement has been performed without significant complication when large particles obtained with a rongeur were used while some hardware failures have been observed with smaller morsels obtained with small rasps bone mills. These clinical observations found their explanation in the lower shear properties of the small particles.

3.1.2.2 The role of fluids

From the soil mechanic theory, it is known that the mechanical strength of a mixture is reduced when too much fluid is present with no drainage possibility, similarly to quicksand (97). The release of excessive fat and marrow that is captured in the closed system may prevent the compactive effort (87). The recoil of smaller bone chips was also significantly higher and increased after impaction with higher force than those from larger chips (95, 98).

Influence of Freeze-Drying and Irradiation on Mechanical Properties of Human Cancellous Bone: Application to Impaction Bone Grafting

49

This might explain why clinicians recommended larger particles rather than slurry (99). The advantage of large morsels on small ones might be tight to the preservation of a trabecular structure and to fat and marrow retention in the interstices (96).

Removing excessive and lubricating fluid of the graft material improved overall graft strength (100-101). While reducing the water content alone had some influence on properties, reducing the fat content improved both the static and dynamic behaviour (102). Processing bone particles with solvents, freeze-drying and irradiation improved the compaction properties and the shear strength of the reconstruction. The improvement in strength was due to an increase in the friction angle and a tighter graft compaction secondary to marrow tissue removal. Washed particles might have little lubrification at the contacts with other particles and therefore friction resistance was increased (103). On the other hand, graft stickiness was advocated to increase interparticulate cohesion (104). The combination of human bone marrow stromal cells with washed allograft to produce a living composite, offered a biological and mechanical advantage over the current gold standard of allograft alone and provided a higher shear strength when compared with allograft alone (105).

Improved results observed with freeze-dried irradiated bone may also be related to an incomplete rehydration. Stickiness between freeze-dried irradiated bone morsels and the impactor was observed during our experiments. Conrad et al found that rehydration could last for longer than one day (33). Impacted freeze-dried irradiated grafts could increase the interlocking effect by increasing their water content. In our study on femoral implant stability in a hip simulator, we observed that implant pull-out was extremely difficult in reconstruction with freeze-dried material compared with frozen one after 1 million cycles and did not result in a shear separation of the graft layers.

3.2 Implant stability

When the initial stability of femoral stem is compared in hip simulator models, cemented hip prosthesis stability within a normal medullar canal was higher than stability of femoral revision with impaction bone grafting (106). More subsidence was found in revision with the impaction technique than with a primary prosthesis (107). In our hip simulator model, a stable reconstruction was achieved with freeze-dried irradiated bone as filling material for impaction bone grafting (108). The stability was even greater than with frozen morsels and compared favourably with stability of primary stem cementation in the same model (109). Taylor considered that the initial mechanical demand was met when the graft was as strong as the endofemoral cancellous bone in a primary prosthesis (110).

The low subsidence registered in our study was about the same as that reported by Karrholm et al. in a clinical study of revisions with impaction technique and non polished stem (85). As in our experimental observation, a considerable amount of migration occurred during the first week after surgery, giving evidence of graft compaction due to patient activity (111). In the clinical cases, the lowest migration registered by radiostereometry was reported by a group who used a mechanical defatting method of the bone (85, 112). The importance of graft compaction has clearly a strong logical appeal and the lack of sufficient compaction is considered as the most likely explanation for substantial migration in clinical situation (85, 113-114).

If implant stability is the first goal, the impaction procedure must be done with energy until the impactors cannot be further driven into the bone (73, 115). This vigorous procedure exposes to fracture that remains one of the major complications of the impaction technique (72, 116-117). Three to five times fewer hammer shocks were needed to impact the freeze-dried irradiated bone correctly, and less energy was needed to compact the material due to its loss of ductility, reducing the risk of per-operative fracture. In our experiments, femoral fracture was associated with a higher subsidence and inducible displacement, which might further increase the risk of loosening. Recently, an innovative vibration-assisted bone-graft compaction system has been tested to reduce peak loads transmitted to the femoral cortex during graft compaction and prevent the risk of intra-operative fracture (118).

3.3 Impacted graft remodelling

Ling pointed out that the initial stability ensures later stability during the remodeling (119). Slooff et al. considered that morselised and impacted graft should be as resistant as a cortical graft and would remodel like a cancellous graft without transient mechanical weakening (120). The concept relies on the cancellous impacted grafts maintaining its volume during remodeling and not being resorbed.

The remodeling of cancellous graft includes a direct new bone deposition along the trabecula whereas resorption proceeds lately within the inner part of the trabecula with no net volume change (21, 23). The morselised and impacted graft is a porous structure and ingrowth of vessels was firstly thought not be impaired (121). In humans, biopsies often revealed mixed areas of living bone and non vital graft (122-127). Remodeled areas were mainly found in load bearing zones (128).

Tagil and Aspenberg demonstrated that impaction slowed down the remodeling (129). They noted that impaction reduced amounts of fat and marrow cells in the compacted graft which support the idea that the squeezing out of the bone marrow from bone will limit the availability of immunogenic cells and the immunogenicity of the impacted bone (72). This is consistent with the benefit of chemical lipid extraction reported in the same model (27). Removal of bone marrow from cancellous bone reduced the immunogenicity as bone marrow cells carry a wider range of transplantation antigens than osteocytes (91, 130).

New living bone is always limited in impacted bone and will appear only in revascularised area, leaving other areas with either non revascularisation or with only a fibrous recolonisation. Tagil and Aspenberg demonstrated that the mechanical properties of an impacted graft were enhanced by coexistence of fibrous tissue that embedded the particles (131). Nevertheless, Schimmel et al. demonstrated in a goat model that, when remodeling was completed and the interface revascularised, a fibrous membrane developed around the cement and the implant became loose (132). This implies that remodeling is not always beneficial and be hazardous for prosthesis longevity. Therefore, mechanical stability is probably more important and essential (133).

4. References

[1] Harris WH, Crothers O, Oh I. Total hip replacement and femoral-head bone-grafting for severe acetabular deficiency in adults. J Bone Joint Surg Am. 1977; 59:752-9.

[2] Pak JH, Paprosky WG, Jablonsky WS, Lawrence JM. Femoral strut allografts in cementless revision total hip arthroplasty. Clin Orthop Relat Res. 1993; 295:172-8.

[3] Head WC, Wagner RA, Emerson RH Jr, Malinin TI. Revision total hip arthroplasty in the deficient femur with a proximal load-bearing prosthesis. Clin Orthop Relat Res. 1994; 298:119-26.

[4] Gross AE, Hutchison CR. Proximal femoral allografts for reconstruction of bone stock in revision hip arthroplasty. Orthopedics. 1998; 21:999-1001.

[5] Kwong LM, Jasty M, Harris WH. High failure rate of bulk femoral head allografts in total hip acetabular reconstructions at 10 years. J Arthroplasty. 1993; 8:341-6.

[6] Jasty M, Harris WH. Salvage total hip reconstruction in patients with major acetabular bone deficiency using structural femoral head allografts. J Bone Joint Surg Br. 1990; 72:63-7.

[7] Shinar AA, Harris WH. Bulk structural autogenous grafts and allografts for reconstruction of the acetabulum in total hip arthroplasty. Sixteen-year-average follow-up. J Bone Joint Surg Am. 1997; 79:159-68.

[8] Slooff TJ, Huiskes R, van Horn J, Lemmens AJ. Bone grafting in total hip replacement for acetabular protrusion. Acta Orthop Scand. 1984; 55:593-6.

[9] Gie GA, Linder L, Ling RS, Simon JP, Slooff TJ, Timperley AJ. Impacted cancellous allografts and cement for revision total hip arthroplasty. J Bone Joint Surg Br. 1993; 75:14-21.

[10] Slooff TJ, Buma P, Schreurs BW, Schimmel JW, Huiskes R, Gardeniers J. Acetabular and femoral reconstruction with impacted graft and cement. Clin Orthop Relat Res. 1996; 324:108-15.

[11] Ling RS. Cemented revision for femoral failure. Orthopedics. 1996; 19:763-4.

[12] Schreurs BW, Slooff TJ, Buma P, Gardeniers JW, Huiskes R. Acetabular reconstruction with impacted morsellised cancellous bone graft and cement. A 10- to 15-year follow-up of 60 revision arthroplasties. J Bone Joint Surg Br. 1998; 80:391-5.

[13] Timperley AJ, Kenny P, Gie GA. Impaction bone grafting on the femoral side. In : Ch Delloye and G Bannister (Eds). Impaction Bone grafting in revision arthroplasty. Marcel Dekker, New York, 2004; 23:323-348.

[14] Henman P, Finlayson D. Ordering allograft by weight: suggestions for the efficient use of frozen bone-graft for impaction grafting. J Arthroplasty. 2000; 15:368-71.

[15] Michaud RJ, Drabu KJ. Bone allograft banking in the United Kingdom. J Bone Joint Surg Br. 1994; 76:350-1.

[16] Galea G, Kopman D, Graham BJ. Supply and demand of bone allograft for revision hip surgery in Scotland. J Bone Joint Surg Br. 1998; 80:595-9.

[17] Norman-Taylor FH, Villar RN. Bone allograft: a cause for concern? J Bone Joint Surg Br. 1997; 79:178-80.

[18] Hart N, Campbell ED, Kartub MG. Bone banking. A cost effective method for establishing a community hospital bone bank. Clin Orthop Relat Res 1986; 206:295-300.

[19] Palmer SH, Gibbons CL, Athanasou NA. The pathology of bone allograft. J Bone Joint Surg Br. 1999; 81:333-5.

[20] Deijkers RL, Bloem RM, Petit PL, Brand R, Vehmeyer SB, Veen MR. Contamination of bone allografts: analysis of incidence and predisposing factors. J Bone Joint Surg Br. 1997; 7 9:161-6.

[21] Boyce T, Edwards J, Scarborough N. Allograft bone. The influence of processing on safety and performance. Orthop Clin North Am. 1999; 30:571-81.

[22] Jinno T, Miric A, Feighan J, Kirk SK, Davy DT, Stevenson S. The effects of processing and low dose irradiation on cortical bone grafts. Clin Orthop Relat Res. 2000; 375:275-85.

[23] Bright R, Burchardt H. The biomechanical properties of preserved bone grafts. In: Friedlaender G, Mankin H, Sell K (eds). Osteochondral allografts. Boston: Little Brown, 1983: 241-247.

[24] Pelker R, Friedlaender GE, Markham TC. Biomechanical properties of bone allografts. Clin Orthop Relat Res. 1983; 174:54-7.

[25] Conrad EU, Ericksen DP, Tencer AF, Strong DM, Mackenzie AP. The effects of freeze-drying and rehydration on cancellous bone. Clin Orthop Relat Res. 1993; 290:279-84.

[26] Vehmeijer S, Bloem RM. The procurement, processing and preservation of allograft bone. In : Ch Delloye and G Bannister (Eds). Impaction bone grafting in revision arthroplasty. Marcel Dekker, New York, 2004; 3:23-32.

[27] Thoren K, Aspenberg P, Thorngren KG. Lipid extracted bank bone. Bone conductive and mechanical properties. Clin Orthop Relat Res. 1995; 311:232-46.

[28] Triantafyllou N, Sotiropoulos E, Trantafyllou JN. The mechanical properties of the lyophilized and irradiated bone grafts. Acta Orthop Belg 1975; 41(S1): 35-44.

[29] Haut RC, Powlison AC, Rutherford GW, Kateley JR. Order of irradiation and lyophilization on the strength of patellar tendon allografts. Trans Orthop Res Soc 1989; 14:514.

[30] Smith CW, Young IS, Kearney JN. Mechanical properties of tendons: changes with sterilization and preservation. J Biomech Eng. 1996; 118:56-61.

[31] Currey JD. The effects of drying and re-wetting on some mechanical properties of cortical bone. J Biomech. 1988; 21:439-41.

[32] Linde F, Sorensen HC. The effect of different storage methods on the mechanical properties of trabecular bone. J Biomech. 1993; 26:1249-52.

[33] Conrad EU, Ericksen DP, Tencer AF, Strong DM, Mackenzie AP. The effects of freeze-drying and rehydration on cancellous bone. Clin Orthop Relat Res. 1993; 290:279-84.

[34] Cornu O, Banse X, Docquier PL, Luyckx S, Delloye C. Effect of freeze-drying and gamma irradiation on the mechanical properties of human cancellous bone. J Orthop Res. 2000; 18:426-31.

[35] Bright RW, Burstein AH. Material properties of preserved cortical bone. Transact Orthop Res Soc 1978; 3:210.

[36] Vastel L, Meunier A, Siney H, Sedel L, Courpied JP. Effect of different sterilization processing methods on the mechanical properties of human cancellous bone allografts. Biomaterials. 2004; 25:2105-10.

[37] Vastel L, Masse C, Crozier E, Padilla F, Laugier P, Mitton D, Bardonnet R, Courpied JP. Effects of gamma irradiation on mechanical properties of defatted trabecular bone allografts assessed by speed-of-sound measurement. Cell Tissue Bank. 2007; 8:205-10.

[38] Steinhauser E, Diehl P, Hadaller M, Schauwecker J, Busch R, Gradinger R, Mittelmeier W. Biomechanical investigation of the effect of high hydrostatic pressure treatment on the mechanical properties of human bone. J Biomed Mater Res B Appl Biomater. 2006; 76:130-5.

[39] Tosello A. Optimal conditions of gamma type irradiation for inactivating HIV in bone fragments. Consequences in biomechanical resistance of the bone tissue. Chirurgie. 1994; 120:104-6.

[40] Anderson M, Keyak J, Skinner H. Compressive mechanical properties of human cancellous bone after gamma irradiation. J Bone Joint Surg Am. 1992; 74:747-752.

[41] Hamer AJ, Strachan JR, Black MM, Ibbotson CJ, Stockley I, Elson RA. Biochemical properties of cortical allograft bone using a new method of bone strength measurement. A comparison of fresh, fresh-frozen and irradiated bone. J Bone Joint Surg Br. 1996; 78:363-8.

[42] Currey JD, Foreman J, Laketić I, Mitchell J, Pegg DE, Reilly GC. Effects of ionizing radiation on the mechanical properties of human bone. J Orthop Res. 1997; 15:111-7.

[43] Godette GA, Kopta JA, Egle DM. Biomechanical effects of gamma irradiation on fresh frozen allografts in vivo. Orthopedics. 1996; 19:649-53.

[44] Bright RW, Gamble VM, Smarsh JD. Effects of sterilizing irradiation on human bone. In Karatzas P and Triantafyllou N (Eds). Tissue grafts in reconstructive surgery. Greek atomic energy commission, Athens, Greece, 1981; 196-201.

[45] Hamer AJ, Stockley I, Elson RA. Changes in allograft bone irradiated at different temperatures. J Bone Joint Surg Br. 1999; 81:342-4.

[46] Salehpour A, Butler DL, Proch FS, Schwartz HE, Feder SM, Doxey CM, Ratcliffe A. Dose-dependent response of gamma irradiation on mechanical properties and related biochemical composition of goat bone-patellar tendon-bone allografts. J Orthop Res. 1995; 13:898-906.

[47] Mitchell EJ, Stawarz AM, Kayacan R, Rimnac CM. The effect of gamma radiation sterilization on the fatigue crack propagation resistance of human cortical bone. J Bone Joint Surg Am. 2004; 86:2648-57.

[48] Ohan MP, Dunn MG. Glucose stabilizes collagen sterilized with gamma irradiation. J Biomed Mater Res 2003; 67:1188-95.

[49] Akkus O, Belaney RM, Das P. Free radical scavenging alleviates the biomechanical impairment of gamma radiation sterilized bone tissue. J Orthop Res. 2005; 23:838-45.

[50] Drozdz M, Piwowarczyk B, Olczyk K. Effects of ionizing radiation on the content of total collagen and its fractions and the activity of collagenolytic enzymes in rat tissues. Med Pr. 1981; 32:317-22.

[51] Nguyen H, Morgan DA, Forwood MR. Sterilization of allograft bone: effects of gamma irradiation on allograft biology and biomechanics. Cell Tissue Bank. 2007; 8:93-105.

[52] Marzec E. Temperature variation of the relaxation time of alpha-dispersion for gamma-irradiated collagen. Int J Biol Macromol. 1995; 17:3-6.

[53] Grieb TA, Forng RY, Stafford RE, Lin J, Almeida J, Bogdansky S, Ronholdt C, Drohan WN, Burgess WH. Effective use of optimized, high dose gamma irradiation for pathogen inactivation of human bone allografts. Biomaterials 2005; 26:2033-2042.

[54] Dziedzic-Goclawska A, Ostrowski K, Stachowicz W, Michalik J, Grzesik W. Effect of radiation sterilization on the osteoinductive properties and the rate of remodeling of bone implants preserved by lyophilization and deep-freezing. Clin Orthop Relat Res 1991; 272:30-37.

[55] Toritsuka Y, Shino K, Horibe S, Nakamura N, Matsumoto N, Ochi TJ. Effect of freeze-drying or gamma-irradiation on remodeling of tendon allograft in a rat model. J Orthop Res. 1997; 15:294-300.

[56] Wheeler DL, Enneking WF. Allograft bone decreases in strength in vivo over time. Clin Orthop Relat Res. 2005; 435:36-42.

[57] Aspenberg P, Thorén K. Lipid extraction enhances bank bone incorporation. An experiment in rabbits. Acta Orthop Scand. 1990; 61:546-8.

[58] Hannink G, Schreurs BW, Buma P. Irradiation has no effect on the incorporation of impacted morselized bone: a bone chamber study in goats. Acta Orthop Scand 2007; 78:31-8.

[59] Moreau MF, Gallois Y, Basle MF, Chappard D. Gamma irradiation of human bone allografts alters medullary lipids and releases toxic compounds for osteoblast-like cells. Biomaterials 2000; 21:369-376.

[60] Crawford MJ, Swenson CL, Arnoczky SP, O'Shea J, Ross H. Lyophilization does not inactivate infectious retrovirus in systemically infected bone and tendon allografts. Am J Sports Med. 2004; 32:580-6.

[61] Campbell DG, Li P, Stephenson AJ, Oakeshott RD. Sterilization of HIV by gamma irradiation. A bone allograft model. Int Orthop. 1994; 18:172-6.

[62] Conway B, Tomford W, Mankin HJ, Hirsch MS, Schooley RT. Radiosensitivity of HIV-1. Potential application to sterilization of bone allografts. AIDS 1991; 5:608-609.

[63] Hernigou P, Marce D, Juliéron A, Marinello G, Dormont D. Stérilisation osseuse par irradiation et virus VIH. Rev Chir Orthop 1993; 79:445-451.

[64] Fideler B, Vangness T, Moore T, Li Z, Rasheed S. Effects of gamma irradiation on the human immunodeficiency virus. A study in frozen human bone-patellar ligament-bone grafts obtained from infected cadavera. J Bone Joint Surg Am. 1994; 76:1032-1035.

[65] Campbell DG, Li P. Sterilization of HIV with irradiation: relevance to infected bone allografts. Aust N Z J Surg. 1999; 69:517-21.

[66] Hiemstra H, Tersmette M, Vos AH, Over J,Van Berkel MP, De Bree H. Inactivation of human immunodeficiency virus by gamma irradiation and its effects on plasma and coagulation factors. Transfusion 1991; 31:32-39.

[67] Conrad EU, Gretch DR, Obermeyer KR, Moogk MS, Sayers M, Wilson JJ, Strong DM. Transmission of the hepatitis-C virus by tissue transplantation. J Bone Joint Surg Am. 1995; 77:214-24.

[68] Pruss A, Kao M, Gohs U, Koscielny J, von Versen R, Pauli G. Effect of gamma irradiation on human cortical bone transplants contaminated with enveloped and non-enveloped viruses. Biologicals. 2002; 30:125-33.

[69] Simonds RJ, Holmberg SD, Hurwitz RL, Coleman TR, Bottenfield S, Conley LJ, Kohlenberg SH, Castro KG, Dahan BA, Schable CA, et al. Transmission of human immunodeficiency virus type 1 from a seronegative organ and tissue donor. N Engl J Med. 1992; 326:726-32.

[70] Grieb TA, Forng RY, Bogdansky S, Ronholdt C, Parks B, Drohan WN, Burgess WH, Lin J. High-dose gamma irradiation for soft tissue allografts: High margin of safety with biomechanical integrity. J Orthop Res. 2006; 24:1011-8.

[71] . Dormont D. Creutzfeldt-Jakob disease and transplantation: facts and fables. Transplant Proc. 1996; 28:2931-3.

[72] Forsell J. Irradiation of musculoskeletal tissues. In: Tomford W (ed.) Musculoskeletal tissue banking. New-York: Raven, 1993: 149-180.

[73] M. Anastasescou, O. Cornu, Ch. Delloye, J. Gigi . Contamination rate and logarithmic reduction of bacteria by processing of freeze-dried cancellous bone. 3d congress of the European Federation of National Associations of Orthopaedics and Traumatology (EFORT), 6th annual meeting of EAMST, Barcelona, Spain, 23 April 1997.

[74] Anglen J, Apostoles PS, Christensen G, Gainor B, Lane J. Removal of surface bacteria by irrigation. J Orthop Res. 1996; 14:251-4.

[75] Salmela PM, Hirn MY, Vuento RE. The real contamination of femoral head allografts washed with pulse lavage. Acta Orthop Scand. 2002; 73:317-20.

[76] Scarborough NL, White EM, Hughes JV, Manrique AJ, Poser JW. Allograft safety: viral inactivation with bone demineralization. Contemp Orthop. 1995; 31:257-61.

[77] Swenson CL, Arnoczky SP. Demineralization for inactivation of infectious retrovirus in systemically infected cortical bone: in vitro and in vivo experimental studies. J Bone Joint Surg Am. 2003; 85:323-32

[78] Feinstone SM, Mihalik KB, Kamimura T, Alter HJ, London WT, Purcell RH. Inactivation of hepatitis B virus and non-A, non-B hepatitis by chloroform. Infect Immun. 1983; 41:816-21.

[79] World Health Organization. Report of a WHO consultation on public health issues related to animal and human spongiform encephalopathies. WHO/CDS/VPH/92.104, 1992.

[80] Fages J, Poirier B, Barbier Y, Frayssinet P, Joffret ML, Majewski W, Bonel G, Larzul D. Viral inactivation of human bone tissue using supercritical fluid extraction. ASAIO J. 1998; 44:289-93.

[81] Cornu O, Bavadekar A, Godts B, Van Tomme J, Delloye C, Banse X. Impaction bone grafting with freeze-dried irradiated bone. Part II. Changes in stiffness and compactness of morselized grafts: experiments in cadavers. Acta Orthop Scand. 2003; 74:553-8.

[82] Cornu O, Libouton X, Naets B, Godts B, Van Tomme J, Delloye C, Banse X. Freeze-dried irradiated bone brittleness improves compactness in an impaction bone grafting model. Acta Orthop Scand. 2004; 75:309-14.

[83] Cornu O, Manil O, Godts B, Naets B, Van Tomme J, Delloye C, Banse X. Neck fracture femoral heads for impaction bone grafting: evolution of stiffness and compactness

during impaction of osteoarthrotic and neck-fracture femoral heads. Acta Orthop Scand. 2004; 75:303-8.

[84] Carter DR, Hayes WC. The compressive behaviour of bone as a two-phase porous structure. J Bone Joint Surg Am. 1977; 59:954-962.

[85] Karrholm J, Hultmark P, Carlsson L, Malchau H. Subsidence of a non-polished stem in revisions of the hip using impaction allograft. Evaluation with radiostereometry and dual-energy X-ray absorptiometry. J Bone Joint Surg Br. 1999; 81:135-42.

[86] Keaveny TM, Wachtel EF, Guo XE, Hayes WC. Mechanical behavior of damaged trabecular bone. J Biomech 1994; 27:1309-1318.

[87] Dunlop DG, Brewster NT, Madabhushi SP, Usmani AS, Pankaj P, Howie CR. Techniques to improve the shear strength of impacted bone graft: the effect of particle size and washing of the graft. J Bone Joint Surg Am. 2003; 85:639-46.

[88] Höstner J, Hultmark P, Kärrholm J, Malchau H, Tveit M. Impaction technique and graft treatment in revisions of the femoral component : laboratory studies and clinical validation. J Arthroplasty 2001; 16:76-82.

[89] Ullmark G. Bigger size and defatting of bone chips will increase cup stability. Arch Orthop Trauma Surg 2000; 120:445-447.

[90] Carter DR, Spengler DM. Mechanical properties and composition of cortical bone. Clin Orthop Relat Res 1978; 135:192-217.

[91] Davy DT. Biomechanical issues in bone transplantation. Orthop Clin North Am 1999; 30:553-563.

[92] Brewster NT, Gillespie WJ, Howie CR, Madabhushi SP, Usmani AS, Fairbairn DR. Mechanical considerations in impaction bone grafting. J Bone Joint Surg Br 1999; 81:118-124.

[93] Brodt MD, Swan CC, Brown TD. Mechanical behaviour of human morselized cancellous bone in triaxial compression testing. J Orthop Res 1998; 16:43-49.

[94] Giesen EB, Lamerigts NM, Verdonschot N, Buma P, Schreurs BW, Huiskes R. Mechanical characteristics of impacted morsellised bone grafts used in revision of total hip arthroplasty. J Bone Joint Surg Br 1999; 81:1052-1057.

[95] Ullmark G, Nilsson O. Impacted corticocancellous allografts : recoil and strength. J Arthroplasty 1999; 14:1019-1023.

[96] Dunlop DG. Mechanical and biological aspects of impaction bone grafting in revision surgery and the use of a new synthetic bone graft. Thesis, University of Edinburgh, Edinburgh, 2001.

[97] Degoutte G, Royet P. Aide mémoire de mécanique des sols. Publications de l'ENGREF, Aix en Provence, France, 2005.

[98] Kuiper JH, Richardson J. Stability of impaction-grafted hip and knee prostheses: Surgical technique, implant design and graft compaction. In : Ch Delloye and G Bannister (Eds). Impaction bone grafting in revision arthroplasty. Marcel Dekker, New York, 2004; 7:75-94.

[99] Gie GA, Linder L, Ling RS, Simon JP, Slooff TJ, Timperley AJ. Contained morselized allograft in revision total hip arthroplasty. Surgical technique. Orthop Clin North Am 1993; 24:717-725.

[100] Dunlop DG, Howie CR, Madabhushi SP, Usmani AS. Factors influencing impacted bone strength: to wash or not to wash? J Bone Joint Surg Br 2000; 82(S1):78.

[101] Fosse L, Rønningen H, Benum P, Sandven RB. Influence of water and fat content on compressive stiffness properties of impacted morsellized bone: an experimental ex vivo study on bone pellets. Acta Orthop Scand 2006; 77:15-22.

[102] Voor MJ, Nawab A, Malkani AL, Ullrich CR. Mechanical properties of compacted morselized cancellous bone graft using one-dimensional consolidation testing. J Biomech. 2000; 33:1683-8.

[103] Dunlop D. Impaction bone grafting. A mechanical appraisal with reference to soil engineering. In : Ch Delloye and G Bannister (Eds). Impaction bone grafting in revision arthroplasty. Marcel Dekker, New York, 2004; 6:57-74.

[104] Vehmeijer S, Bloem RM. The procurement, processing and preservation of allograft bone. In : Ch Delloye and G Bannister (Eds). Impaction bone grafting in revision arthroplasty. Marcel Dekker, New York, 2004; 3:23-32.

[105] Bolland BJ, Partridge K, Tilley S, New AM, Dunlop DG, Oreffo RO. Biological and mechanical enhancement of impacted allograft seeded with human bone marrow stromal cells: potential clinical role in impaction bone grafting. Regen Med. 2006; 1:457-67.

[106] Eldridge JD, Smith EJ, Hubble MJ, Whitehouse SL, Learmonth ID. Massive early subsidence following femoral impaction grafting. J Arthroplasty 1997; 12:535-540.

[107] Malkani AR, Voor MJ, Fee KA, Bates CS. Femoral component revisions using impacted morsellized cancellous graft. J Bone Joint Surg Br. 1996; 78:973-978.

[108] Cornu O, Bavadekar A, Godts B, Van Tomme J, Delloye C, Banse X. Impaction bone grafting with freeze-dried irradiated bone. Part I. Femoral implant stability: cadaver experiments in a hip simulator. Acta Orthop Scand. 2003; 74:547-52.

[109] Godts B, Bavadekar A, Cornu O, Verhelpen M, Delloye Ch. Comparative dynamic loading of paired femurs. Comparison of freeze-dried versus fresh-frozen bone allografts. In : Ch Delloye and G Bannister (Eds). Impaction bone grafting in revision arthroplasty. Marcel Dekker, New York, 2004; 12:157-176.

[110] Taylor M, Tanner KE. Fatigue failure of cancellous bone: a possible cause of implant migration and loosening. J Bone Joint Surg Br. 1997; 79:181-182.

[111] Ornstein E, Franzen H, Johnsson R, Sundberg M. Radiostereometric analysis in hip revision surgery: optimal time for index examination. 6 patients revised with impacted allografts and cement followed weekly for 6 weeks. Acta Orthop Scand 2000; 71:360-364.

[112] Nivbrant B, Kärrholm J. Increased subsidence of uncemented femoral stems in hip revisions with impaction bone grafting. Acta Orthop Scand 1997; 274(S1):79-80.

[113] Franzen H, Toksvig-Larsen S, Lidgren L, Önnerfält R. Early migration of femoral component revised with impacted cancellous allografts and cement. A preliminary report of five patients. J Bone Joint Surg Am. 1995; 77:862-864.

[114] Masterson EL, Duncan CP. Subsidence and the cement mantle in femoral impaction allografting. Orthopedics 1997; 20:821-822.

[115] Schreurs BW, Gardeniers JW, Slooff TJ. Acetabular reconstruction with bone impaction grafting: 20 years of experience. Instr Course Lect. 2001; 50:221-8.

[116] Leopold SS, Jacobs JJ, Rosenberg AG. Cancellous allograft in revision total hip arthroplasty. A clinical review. Clin Orthop Relat Res 2000; 371:86-97.

[117] Pekkarinen J, Alho A, Lepisto J, Ylikoski M, Ylinen P, Paavilainen T. Impaction bone grafting in revision hip surgery. A high incidence of complications. J Bone Joint Surg Br. 2000; 82:103-107.

[118] Bolland BJ, New AM, Madabhushi SP, Oreffo RO, Dunlop DG. Vibration-assisted bone-graft compaction in impaction bone grafting of the femur. J Bone Joint Surg Br. 2007; 89:686-92.

[119] Ling RSM. Femoral component revision using impacted morsellized cancellous graft. J Bone Joint Surg Br. 1997; 79:874-880.

[120] Slooff TJ, Schimmel JW, Buma P. Cemented fixation with bone grafts.Orthop Clin North Am. 1993; 24:667-77.

[121] Stevenson S. Enhancement of fracture healing with autogenous and allogenic bone grafts. Clin Orthop Relat Res 1998; 355:239-246.

[122] Ling RS, Timperley AJ, Linder L. Histology of cancellous impaction grafting in the femur. A case report. J Bone Joint Surg Br. 1993; 75:693-696.

[123] Nelissen RG, Weidenhielm LR, LeGolvan DP, Mikhail WE. Revision hip arthroplasty with the use of cement and impaction bone grafting. Histological analysis of four cases. J Bone Joint Surg Am. 1995; 77:412-422.

[124] Heekin RD, Engh CA, Vinh T. Morselized allograft in acetabular reconstruction. A post-mortem retrieval analysis. Clin Orthop Relat Res 1995; 319:184-190.

[125] Buma P, Lamerigts N, Schreurs BW, Gardeniers J, Versleyen D, Slooff TJ. Impacted graft incorporation after cemented acetabular revision. Histological evaluation in 8 patients. Acta Orthop Scand 1996; 67:536-540.

[126] Ullmark G, Linder L. Histology of the femur after cancellous imaction bone grafting using Charnley prosthesis. Arch Orthop Trauma Surg 1998; 117:170-172.

[127] Whiteside LA, Bicalho PS. Radiologic and histologic analysis of morselised allograft in revision total knee replacement. Clin Orthop Relat Res 1998; 357:149-156.

[128] Linder L, Ling RSM, Gie GA, Timperley AJ. Histological analysis of cancellous impaction grafting in the femur: a retrieval study of five human femora. In: proceedings Am Acad Orthop Surg, New Orleans, USA 1998:185.

[129] Tägil M, Aspenberg P. Impaction of cancellous bone grafts impairs osteoconduction in titanium chambers in rats. Clin Orthop Relat Res 1998; 352:231-238.

[130] Richards RR, Langer F, Halloran P, Gross AE. The antigenic profile of the immune skeletal system. Trans Orthop Res Soc 1979; 4:79.

[131] Tägil M, Aspenberg P. Fibrous tissue armouring increases the mechanical strength of an impacted bone graft. Acta Orthop Scand 2001; 72:78-82.

[132] Schimmel JW, Buma P, Versleyen D, Huiskes R, Slooff TJ. Acetabular reconstruction with impacted morselized cancellous allografts in cemented hip arthroplasty: a histological and biomechanical study on the goat. J Arthroplasty. 1998; 13:438-48.

[133] Linder L. Cancellous impaction bone grafting in the human femur. Acta Orthop Scand 2000; 71:543-552.

Part 3

Trauma Surgery

4

Reconstruction of Post-Traumatic Bone Defect of the Upper-Limb with Vascularized Fibular Graft

R. Adani[1], L. Tarallo[2] and R. Mugnai[2]
[1]Hand and Microsurgery Department, Policlinico GB Rossi,
Azienda Ospedaliera Universitaria Verona, Verona,
[2]Department of Orthopaedic Surgery,
University of Modena and Reggio Emilia, Policlinico di Modena, Modena,
Italy

1. Introduction

Fracture non-union or delayed union frequently occur after high-energy traumas associated to significant bony tissue loss, in open fractures with infections, and after an inappropriate use of internal fixation.[1,2,3,4,5,6,7] Obesity, smoking, abuse of alcohol or drugs, osteoporosis and immunodepression are additional factors that prevent bone healing.[1,4,6] Based on characteristic of the bone ends, non-unions may be atrophic, oligotrophic, and hypertrophic.[8,9,10] Atrophic non-unions have little or no callus formation and are often characterized by bone resorption with normal healing, being limited by inadequate biological response at the fracture site. In turn, in oligotrophic and hypertrophic non-unions the blood supplies are adequate and abundant calluses are seen. In this case, the main reason for the non-union is an insufficient mechanical stability. Generally, the majority of non-unions are atrophic.[11,12,13]

A number of surgical options for the treatment of upper limb bony non-union, including intramedullary nailing,[2,14,15] distraction with an Ilizarov fixator,[4,16,17,18,19] and plate compression with or without conventional bone grafting,[6,20] have been described over the years. The use of these therapeutic options achieves bony union in 82% to 95% of patients.[4] Causes of unsuccessful outcomes can be the result of inadequate techniques of osteosynthesis with unsatisfactory stabilization or with persistence of infection, but failure mostly occur in bony defects greater than 6 cm.[21,22] Bone grafts and bone graft substitutes have a number of inherent properties that allow them to initiate, stimulate, and facilitate bony healing.[23,24] (Table 1) Osteoconduction refers to the process by which the graft provides a scaffold for the ordered 3-D ingrowth of capillaries, perivascular tissue, and osteoprogenitor cells. Osteoinduction refers to the recruitment of osteoprogenitor cells from surrounding tissue. Osteogenesis refers to the formation of new bone from either the host or graft tissue. In addition to these three properties, it is important to consider the mechanical strength and vascularity of the bone graft material. Autogenous and allogenic cortical and cancellous bone grafts are all, to varying degrees, osteoconductive, osteoinductive, and osteogenic. For these reasons, non-vascularized bone grafts are effective in facilitating bony healing. When properly utilized, non-vascularized bone grafts may be incorporated into the adjacent host bone through the process of "creeping substitution". The bone graft material, through the invasion of capillaries, perivascular tissue, and inflammatory cells, is gradually revascularized and ultimately resorbed, allowing for the formation of new living bone which is incorporated and remodeled into the host skeleton. However, this process takes time, during which the structural integrity and mechanical strength of the bone graft and host bone may be impaired23 Autograft is the most commonly used type of bone graft.[25] It can come from a variety of areas, including the iliac crest, distal femur, proximal tibia, fibula, distal radius, and olecranon. Nonvascularized iliac crest bone grafts are effective in the management of defects smaller than 5 to 6 cm in length in the presence of well-perfused soft tissue with no active infection.[26] The use of nonvascularized fibular grafts has provided interesting results;[8,27] however, this technique requires a prolonged immobilization and a consolidation time ranging between 6-11 months.[28] In addition, bone allografts do not yeld satisfactory results if the recipient site is not well vascularized or if infection is present.[29] Vascularized bone grafts, by definition, are placed with their vascularity intact, and thus are immediately viable. As a result, vascularized bone grafts obviate the need for incorporation by creeping substitution and may instead incorporate into the adjacent host bone via primary (or secondary) bone healing. This process allows for the mechanical strength and structural integrity of the vascularized graft to be preserved, which may provide greater strength and more immediate stability to the recipient site. Vascularized bone transfer are more efficient than conventional corticocancellous interposition grafting for the management of massive bone loss (>6 cm).[30,31] Vascularized bone grafting has several advantages in the treatment of non-union,[32] in particular the living bone graft can provide osteogenic cells, improve vascularity at the bone junction, eliminate infection and enhance the intrinsic stability at the site of non-union, thereby permitting simpler and more rapid fracture healing.[33]

Type of Graft	Osteoconduction	Osteoinduction	Osteogenesis	Mechanical strength	Vascularity
Bone Marrow	+/-	+	++	-	-
Cancellous autograft	++	+	++	+	-
Cortical autograft	+	+/-	+	++	-
Vascularized	++	+	++	++	++

Table 1. Properties of bone grafts

2. Vascularized fibular graft

Almost 30 years have elapsed since the vascularized fibula graft was first mentioned in the literature,[34] and this technique is now commonly used in clinical practice. Biomechanically, the fibula bears only 15 percent of the axial load across the ankle, allowing for its use as an autogenous bone graft with minimal biomechanical consequences on the weight-bearing status of the lower limb.[35] As also the distal fibula plays an important role in conferring rotational stability and restraint against lateral translation of the talus, efforts are made to preserve the distal fibula during graft harvest to avoid subsequent ankle deformity or instability.[36,37,38] The vascular supply to the fibula has been well established.[34,38] The endosteal blood supply to the fibula is provided by a nutrient artery which typically enters the posterior fibular cortex at the junction of the proximal one-third and distal two-thirds. This nutrient artery is a branch of the peroneal artery, which runs along the posterior aspect of the fibular diaphysis. The peroneal artery arises from the posterior tibial artery approximately 2 to 3 cm below the lower border of the popliteus muscle, it passes towards the fibula and descends along its medial border, between tibialis posterior and flexor hallucis longus and divides into calcaneal branches which ramify on the lateral and posterior surfaces of the calcaneum. These vessels anastomose with the anterior and posterior tibial. The peroneal artery supplies the nutrient vessels to the fibula which enter on the posteromedial surface of the bone. At approximately 2 to 5 cm intervals throughout its length, septocutaneous vessels arise, which pass laterally, sometimes through the edge of soleus, onto the posterior surface of the lateral intermuscular septum.[39] The fibula free flap based on the peroneal artery and its venae comitantes lies medial to the fibula and posterior to the interosseous membrane. Based upon this understanding of the vascularity of the fibula, techniques of vascularized fibula graft harvest, which preserve both the nutrient artery and the rich periosteal blood supply, have been developed. The use of vascularized fibular graft in reconstructive surgery of the upper extremity was introduced at the end of the 1970s,[40] and for a long time its application in posttraumatic reconstruction of the forearm was limited to a small number of isolated clinical cases.[31,41,42,43,44,45] In 1984, Dell and Sheppard described its use in the treatment of infected pseudoarthrosis of the forearm, and reported on 4 cases.[46] It was not until 1991 that a significant series was reported in the literature;[47] some other papers were recently published on this subject.[29,48,49,50,51,52,53] With advancements in microsurgical techniques, vascularized bone grafts have become well-established technical resources capable of providing solutions to difficult reconstructive challenges.[32] The use of free fibula flap in the treatment of upper limb diaphyseal non-unions has also gained increased popularity over the last few decades. The reason for this are (1) increased vascularity at the fracture site is essential in promoting a faster bone healing and fighting infection and (2) vascularized bone provides higher biomechanical strength than nonvascularized bone.[29] Vascularized fibular grafting also has a number of additional theoretical advantages over conventional, non-vascularized bone grafting techniques. Given the length of fibular diaphysis that may be harvested, free fibular grafts are well suited for the reconstruction of segmental defects of the long bones, providing both mechanical strength and biological stimulus for healing. Furthermore, based upon the fasciocutaneous arterial branches of the peroneal artery, skin, fascia, and muscle may be harvested concomitantly with the fibula to allow for more complex soft tissue reconstruction. Moreover, given the ability to transfer the proximal fibular epiphysis with the diaphysis during free vascularized fibular grafting, there is potential for preserving continued skeletal growth of the fibular graft.[54] Finally, the fibula is a long and straight tubular bone, which is not difficult to harvest, while donor site morbidity is minimal up to a graft length of 20 cm.[55,56] The anatomy is predictable, and its size and shape allows a satisfactory fixation of femoral, tibial, and humeral defects.[55,56] Free fibula flap in long bones reconstruction is an useful and versatile procedure for defects greater than 6-8 cm.[29,32,57,58] It has been demonstrated that, when appropriate blood perfusion is restored to the flap, the proximal and distal fracture sites have the same healing potential of a bifocal fracture with no bone tissue loss, and with no vascular impairment to the central segment. Despite its many theoretical advantages and applications, however, free vascularized fibula grafting is technically challenging and confers its own set of inherent risks and potential complications. Sound microsurgical technique is essential in performing the required arterial and venous anastamoses and ensuring long-term graft viability. Furthermore, donor site morbidity has been well documented, and up to 10% of patients may subsequently develop ankle pain, instability, and/or progressive valgus deformity if fibula harvest is not performed with a proper technique.[59,60] Given these considerations, free vascularized fibula grafting should be employed in specific clinical situations. Presently, the indications for free vascularized fibula grafting fall into two categories.[61] (Table 2) The former is for segmental bony defects greater than 6 to 8 cm, such as those seen in post-traumatic or post-infectious bone loss and tumor resection. The latter is for smaller bony defects in which a biological failure of bony healing, such as those seen in recalcitrant fracture non unions, congenital pseudarthroses, and osteonecrosis, has occurred. Accurate patient selection with a careful clinical evaluation is essential in order to reduce the complication rate. Chronic infections, diabetes, immunosoppression, alcohol, tobacco, drug abuse and obesity are relative contraindications to the procedure. Furthermore, the local wound conditions, the trauma etiology and the outcome of previous surgeries should also be carefully considered.[55] The fibula may be used as graft material in the cervical spine, clavicle, humerus, radius, ulna, lumbar spine, femur (including knee arthrodesis), tibia, and ankle. In the shoulder, the free fibula graft may be used to augment arthrodesis or to treat the patient with prosthesis failure and massive bone loss.[62] In the humerus, fibula graft can be used to manage non-union, infection, and epiphyseal fracture. Fibula graft can be used to manage radius and ulna defects or in creating a one-bone forearm. The overall success rate of the procedure, estimated from the literature, varies from 76% to 100%, with a healing time ranging from 3.7 to 8.9 months.[63] In a large Mayo cohort, the primary and secondary union rates in vascularized fibular grafts performed for non-osteomyelitis indications were 69% and 84%, respectively, but in series of defects with infections, the union rates fall to 49% and 77%.[64] From a meta-analysis of 13 different series involving 317 reconstructions for atrophic non-unions, the mean time for fracture consolidation appeared to be 5.5 months in the 87% of patients.[22] In cases of severely injured limb complicated by infection and large bony defects, the success rate of reconstruction was lowered to 71.5%.[65] In a research we performed on forearm non-union with a bony defect ranging from 6 cm to 13 cm, treated with vascularized fibular graft, the complete healing was obtained in 11/12 cases, with a mean period for radiographic bony union of 4.8 months.[52] A review of the available literature shows only a few reports of vascularized bone grafting for non-union of the humeral shaft. Jupiter reported 4 patients, and 3 of them went to primary bony union within 4 months.[1] Muramatsu et al. reported 9 patients with recalcitrant non-union of the humerus reconstructed by a vascularized fibular graft, and the mean time for union was 6 months (range, 4-10 months).[4] The results of our previous research did not differ very much from these reports: our mean healing time was 6 months (range, 3-13 months) in a series of 13 cases with bony defect ranging from 6 to 16 cm.[53] Among different possible complications, stress fractures of the graft represent a possible event. Vascularized bone grafts have decreased the incidence of stress fractures with respect to conventional bone grafts;[64] their incidence is reported in 15% to 20% of cases.[2,52,58,65,66] Most fracture occurs within the first year of surgery, when the bone has insufficient time to hypertrophy.[64,67] Therefore, de Boer et al. recommend that a vascularized graft should be protected against stress fracture during the first year, allowing for a gradual increase in mechanical loading that enhances remodeling and hypertrophy.[68] Other complications associated with the procedure are secondary infection, delayed union, recurrent non-union, transient palsy of the radial nerve, and vascular impairment to the pedicle flap. These complications occur in 7% to 10% of cases.[65] Complications to the donor site are rare, however they may include peroneal palsy, contracture of the long flexor tendon of the great toe, compartment syndrome in the lower limb, valgus deformity of the ankle, or even a spontaneous fracture of the ipsilateral tibia.[69,70]

	Traumatic bone loss
Segmental bone defects greater than 6 – 8 cm	Tumor resection
	Osteonecrosis
	Osteomyelitis
	Persistent non-union
Biological failure of bony healing	Infected non-union
	Congenital pseudarthrosis

Table 2. Indications for free vascularized fibula grafting

3. Surgical technique

A brief description of the technique of free vascularized fibula graft harvest is provided to give the reader some insight on related surgical considerations and applications. Preoperative planning for vascularized fibula transfer involves coordination of recipient vessels, bone length, and internal fixation. Recipient vessels must be large enough in diameter to accept the peroneal artery, which can be quite large in adults.[71] One artery and two veins are preferred as recipient vessels. For vascular access, the brachial artery or distal branching into the radial artery can be used for inflow, particularly around the humerus. An existing end artery from previous trauma resection in the upper extremity should be used as an end-to-end anastomosis. When the fibula is to be harvested without accompanying skin or soft-tissue, a longitudinal incision is made over the lateral aspect of the fibula. Superficial dissection is performed in the interval between the peroneus longus muscle anteriorly and the soleus posteriorly. The diaphysis of the fibula is then circumferentially exposed with care being made to preserve the periosteum and periosteal blood supply; this results in the typical "marbled" appearance to the fibular graft. Circumferential dissection of the fibula is continued anteriorly and posteriorly, reflecting the peroneal and flexor hallucis longus muscles, respectively. The peroneal artery and vein are identified along the posterior aspect of the fibula and carefully protected as the intermuscular septum is divided along the length of the proposed graft. The fibula is osteotomized proximally and distally, with preservation of the peroneal vessels. Once the recipient site is prepared, the vascular pedicle may be divided and the fibula transferred to the desired location. If an osteomyocutaneous flap is required, dissection starts with a linear lateral incision over the fibula paralleling to its border. The skin paddle is centered over the distal one third of the flap as most cutaneous perforators will arise in the distal half of the lower leg. The skin paddle is incised and elevated in a subfascial plane over the peroneus longus and brevis muscles anteriorly and the soleus and gastrocnemius muscles posteriorly. Dissection is continued until the posterior intermuscular septum is reached. At this point, septocutaneous perforators passing into the skin paddle are identified. Only one perforator is required, but as many as possible of them are included in the dissection. If no such perforators are identified, another reconstructive modality is chosen for the cutaneous portion of the defect, and a bone only fibula flap is harvestened. The peroneus longus and brevis muscles are freed from the anterolateral part of the fibula allowing the access to the interosseous membrane, which is next released. Proximal and distal osteotomies are made in the fibula. The pedicle is than traced proximally to its origin. Once flap harvest has been completed, closure of the leg is accomplished by careful muscle reapproximation and split thickness skin graft application to the donor site. After the stabilization of the fibula to the recipient site, typically done with rigid internal screw fixation, microvascular anastamoses are performed, reconstituting both arterial inflow and venous outflow to the fibular graft. In the figures are briefly reported two cases in which we used the vascularized fibular graft for the treatment of respectively distal humerus (Case 1) and radial diaphysis (Case 2) non-unions.

Case 1. Non-union of the distal humerus

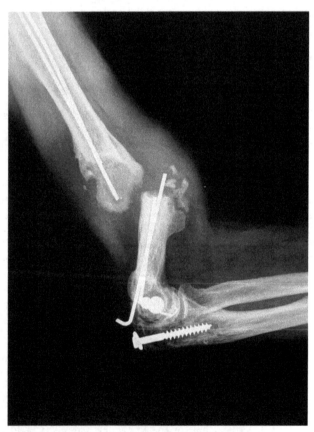

Fig. 1A. Non-union of the distal humerus treated with 2 K.wires

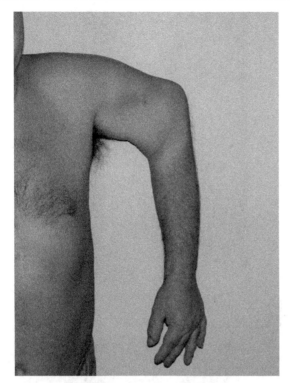

Fig. 1B. Clinic view with a new joint (non-union) upper the elbow

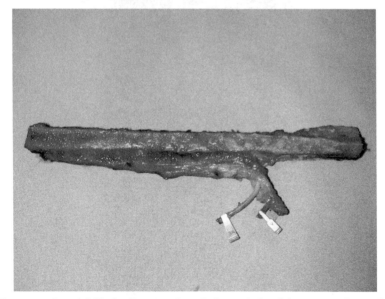

Fig. 1C. Free vascularized fibular bone graft with the pedicle of the peroneal vessels

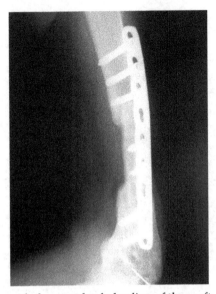

Fig. 1D. Rx after 6 months with the completely healing of the graft

Case 2. Non-union of the radial diaphysis

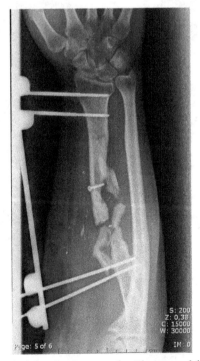

Fig. 2A. Non-union of the radial diaphysis treated with external fixation

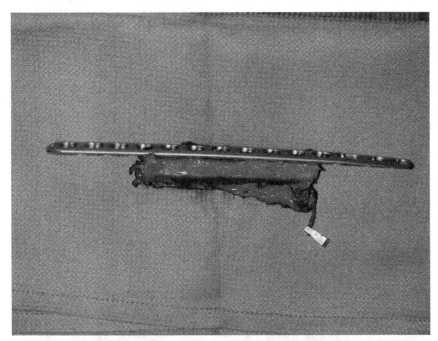

Fig. 2B. Free vascularized fibular bone graft with the pedicle of the peroneal vessels

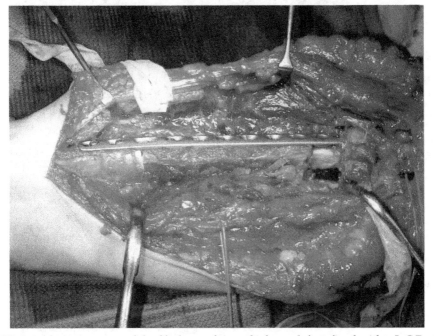

Fig. 2C. Intraoperative view of the fibular graft into the bone defect, fixed with a L.C.P. plate

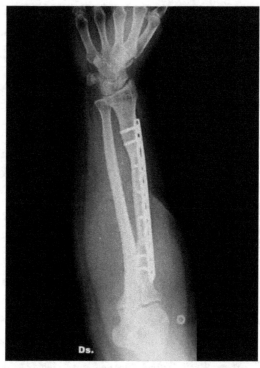

Fig. 2D. Rx after 12 months with the completely healing of the graft

4. References

[1] Jupiter JB. Complex non-union of the humeral diaphysis. Treatment with a medial approach, an anterior plate, and a vascularized fibular graft. J Bone Joint Surg Am 1990;72:701-7.

[2] de Boer HH, Wood MB, Hemans J. Reconstruction of the large skeletal defects by vascularized fibula transfer. Int Orthop 1990;14:121-8.

[3] McKee MD, Miranda MA, Riemer BL, Blasier RB, Redmond BJ, Sims SH, Waddell JP, Jupiter JB. Management of humeral non-union after the failure of locking intramedullary nails. J Orthop Trauma 1996;10:492-9.

[4] Muramatsu K, Doi K, Ihara K, Shigetomi M, Kawai S. Recalcitrant posttraumatic non-union of the humerus. Acta Orthop Scand 2003;74:95-7.

[5] Patel VR, Menon DK, Pool RD, Simonis RB. Non-union of the humerus after failure of surgical treatment. Management using the Ilizarov circular fixation. J Bone Joint Surg Br 2000;82:977-83.

[6] Ring D, Jupiter JB, Quintero J, Sanders RA, Marti RK. Atrophic ununited diaphyseal fractures of the humerus with a bony defect. J Bone Joint Surg Br 2000;82: 867-71.

[7] Volgas DA, Stannard JP, Alonso JE. Non-unions of the humerus. Clin Orthop 2004;419:46-50.

[8] Moroni A, Rollo G, Guzzardella M, Zinghi G. Surgical treatment of isolated forearm non-union with segmental bone loss. Injury 1997;28(8):497-504.

[9] Moroni A, Caja VL, Sbato C, Rollo G, Zinghi G. Composite bone grafting and plate fixation for the treatment of non-unions of the forearm with segmental bone loss: a report of eight cases. J Orthop Trauma 1995;9:419-426.

[10] Naimark A, Miller K, Segal D, Kossoff J. Non-union. Skeletal Radiol 1981;6(1):21-25.

[11] Grace TG, Eversmann WW Jr. The management of segmental bone loss associated with forearm fractures. J Bone Joint Surg Am 1980;62(7):1150-5.

[12] Miller RC, Phalen GS. The repair of defects of the radius with fibular bone grafts. J Bone Joint Surg Am 1947;29:629-36.

[13] Spira E. Bridging of bone defects in the forearm with iliac graft combined with intramedullary nailing. J Bone Joint Surg Br 1954;36:642-6.

[14] Paramasivan ON, Younge DA, Pant R. Treatment of non-union around the olecranon fossa of the humerus by intramedullary locked nail. J Bone Joint Surg Br 2000;82:332-5.

[15] Wu CC. Humeral shaft non-union treated by a Seidel interlocking nail with a supplementary staple. Clin Orthop 1996;326:203-8.

[16] Catagni MA, Guerreschi F, Probe RA. Treatment of humeral non-unions with the Ilizarov technique. Bull Hosp Jt Dis 1991;51:74-83.

[17] Cattaneo R, Catagni MA, Guerreschi F. Applications of the Ilizarov method in the humerus: lengthenings and non-unions. Hand Clin 1993;9:729-39.

[18] Ciuccarelli C, Cervellati C, Montanari G, Masetti G, Galli G, Carpanelli F. The Ilizarov method for the treatment of non-union in the humerus. Chir Organi Mov 1990;75:115-20.

[19] Lammens J, Bauduin G, Dreisen R, Moens P, Stuyck J, De Smet L, Fabry G. Treatment of non-union of the humerus using the Ilizarov external fixator. Clin Orthop 1998;353:223-30.

[20] Trotter DH, Dobozi W. Non-union of the humerus: rigid fixation, bone grafting, and adjunctive bone cement. Clin Orthop 1986;204:62-8.

[21] Heitmann C, Erdmann D, Levin LS. Treatment of segmental defects of the humerus with an osteoseptocutaneous fibular transplant. J Bone Joint Surg Am 2002;84:2216-23.

[22] Tu YK, Yen CH, Yeh WL,Wang IC, Wang KC, Ueng SWN. Reconstruction of posttraumatic long bone defect with free vascularized bone graft: good outcome in 48 patients with 6 years' follow-up. Acta Orhop Scand 2001;72:359-64.

[23] Buckwalter JA, Einhorn TA, Simon SR, eds. Orthopaedic Basic Science. Chicago: American Academy of Orthopaedic Surgeons, 2000.

[24] Khan SN, Cammisa FP, Sandhu HS, Diwan AD, Firardi FP, Lane JM. The biology of bone grafting. J Am Acad Orthop Surg 2005;13:77-86.

[25] Lieberman JR, Daluiski A, Einhorn TA. The role of growth factors in the repair of bone. Biology and clinical applications. J Bone Joint Surg Am 2002;84:1032-1044.

[26] Brunelli GA, Vigasio A, Brunelli GR. Microvascular fibular grafts in skeleton reconstruction. Clin Orthop 1995;314:241-6.

[27] Al Zahrani S, Harding MG, Kremli M, Khan FA, Ikram A, Takroni T. Free fibular graft still has a place in the treatment of bone defects. Injury 1993;24:551-554.

[28] Stevanovic M, Gutow AP, Sharpe F. The management of bone defects of the forearm after trauma. Hand Clin 1999;15:299-318.

[29] Mattar R Jr, Azze RJ, Castro Ferreira M, Starck R, Canedo AC. Vascularized fibular graft for management of severe osteomyelitis of the upper extremity. Microsurgery 1994;15:22-7.

[30] Ruch DS, Weiland AJ, Wolfe SW, Geissler WB, Cohen MS, Jupiter JB. Current concepts in the treatment of distal radial fractures. Instr Course Lect. 2004;53:389-401. Review.

[31] Wood MB. Upper extremity reconstruction by vascularized bone transfers: results and complications. J Hand Surg Am. 1987;12(3):422-7.

[32] Moran CG, Wood MB. Vascularized bone autografts. Orthop Rev 1993;22(2):187-97.

[33] Duffy GP, Wood MB, Rock MG, Sim FH. Vascularized free fibular transfer combined with autografting for the management of fracture non-unions associated with radiation therapy. J Bone Joint Surg Am. 2000;82(4):544-54.

[34] Taylor GI, Miller GDH, Ham FJ. The free vascularized bone graft: a clinical extension of microvascular techniques. Plast Reconstr Surg 1975;55:533-544.

[35] Lambert KL. The weight-bearing function of the fibula. A strain gauge study. J Bone Joint Surg Am 1971;53:507-513.

[36] Pacelli LL, Gillard J, McLoughlin SW, Buehler MJ. A biomechanical analysis of donor-site ankle instability following free fibular graft harvest. J Bone Joint Surg Am 2006;85:597-603.

[37] Vail TP, Urbaniak JR. Donor-site morbidity with the use of vascularized autogenous fibular grafts. J Bone Joint Surg Am 1996;78:204-211.

[38] Malizos KN, Zalavras CG, Soucacos PN, Beris AE, Urbaniak JR. Free vascularized fibular grafts for reconstruction of skeletal defects. J Am Acad Orthop Surg 2004;12:360-369.

[39] Carr AJ, Macdonald DA, Waterhouse N. The blood supply of the osteocutaneous free fibular graft. J Bone Joint Surg Br 1988;70(2):319-21.

[40] Weiland AJ, Kleinert HE, Kutz JE, Daniel RK. Free vascularized bone grafts in surgery of the upper extremity. J Hand Surg Am 1979;4:129-143.

[41] Chuang DC-C, Chen H-C, Wei FC. Compound functioning free muscle flap transplantation (lateral half of soleus, fibula, and skin flap). Plast Reconstr Surg 1992;89:335-339.

[42] Hurst LC, Mirza MA, Spellman W. Vascularized fibular graft for infected loss of the ulna: case report. J Hand Surg Am 1982;7:498-501.

[43] Jones NF, Swartz WM, Mears DC, Jupiter JB, Grossman A. The "double barrel" free vascularized bone graft. Plast Reconstr Surg 1988;81:378-385.

[44] Koshima I, Higaki H, Soeda S. Combined vascularized fibula and peroneal composite-flap transfer for severe heat-press injury of the forearm. Plast Reconstr Surg 1991;88:338-341.

[45] Santanelli F, Latini C, Leanza L, Scuderi N. Combined radius and ulna reconstruction with a free fibula transfer. Br J Plast Surg 1996;49:178-182.

[46] Dell PC, Sheppard JE. Vascularized bone grafts in the treatment of infected forearm non-unions. J Hand Surg Am 1984;9:653-658.

[47] Olekas J, Guobys A. Vascularized bone transfer for defects and pseudoarthrosis of forearm bones. J Hand Surg Br 1991;16:406-408.

[48] Jupiter JB, Gerhard HJ, Guerrero JA, Nunley J, Levin LS. Treatment segmental defects of the radius with use of the vascularized osteoseptocutaneous fibular autogenous graft. J Bone Joint Surg Am 1997;79:542-550.

[49] Tang C-H. Reconstruction of the bones and joints of the upper extremity by vascularized free fibular graft: report of 46 cases. J Reconstr Microsurg 1992;8:285-292.

[50] Yajima H, Tamai S, Ono H, Kizaki K. Vascularized bone grafts to the upper extremities. Plast Reconstr Surg 1998;101:727-735.

[51] Yajima H, Tamai S, Ono H, Kizaki K, Yamauchi T. Free vascularized fibula grafts in surgery of the upper limb. J Reconstr Microsurg 1999;15:515-521.

[52] Adani R, Delcroix L, Innocenti M, Marcoccio I, Tarallo L, Celli A, Ceruso M. Reconstruction of large posttraumatic skeletal defects of the forearm by vascularized free fibular graft. Microsurgery 2004;6:423-9.

[53] Adani R, Delcroix L, Tarallo L, Baccarani A, Innocenti M. Reconstruction of posttraumatic bone defects of the humerus with vascularized fibular graft. J Shoulder Elbow Surg 2008;17(4):578-84.

[54] Tsai TM, Ludwig L, Tonkin M. Vascularized fibular epiphyseal transfer. A clinical study. Clin Orthop Relat Res 1986;210:228-234.

[55] Harrison DH. The osteocutaneous free fibular graft. J Bone Joint Surg Br. 1986;68(5):804-7.

[56] Shalaby S, Shalaby H, Bassiony A. Limb salvage for osteosarcoma of the distal tibia with resection arthrodesis, autogenous fibular graft and Ilizarov external fixator. J Bone Joint Surg Br. 2006;88(12):1642-6.

[57] Gonzàlez del Pino J, Bartolomé del Valle E, Graña GL, Villanova JF. Free vascularized fibula grafts have a high union rate in atrophic non-unions. Clin Orthop 2004;419:38-45.

[58] Minami A, Kasashima T, Iwasaki N, Kato H, Kaneda K. Vascularized fibular grafts: an experience of 102 patients. J Bone Joint Surg Br 2000;82:1022-5.

[59] Vail TP, Urbaniak JR. Donor-site morbidity with the use of vascularized autogenous fibular grafts. J Bone Joint Surg Am 1996;78:204-211.

[60] Kanaya K, Wada T, Kura H, Yamashita T, Usui M, Ishii S. Valgus deformity of the ankle following harvesting of a vascularized fibular graft in children. J Reconstr Microsurg 2002;18:91-96.

[61] Green DP, Hotchkiss RN, Pederson WC, Wolfe S, eds. Green's Operative Hand Surgery, 5th ed. Philadelphia: Churchill Livingston, 2005.

[62] Levin LS: The use of the osteoseptocutaneous free fibula transfer in the upper extremity, in Reconstructive Microsurgery [DVD]. Rosemont, IL: American Society for Surgery of the Hand, 1996.

[63] Lee KS, Park JW. Free vascularized osteocutaneous fibular graft to the tibia. Microsurgery 1999;19:141-7.

[64] Han CS, Wood MB, Bishop AT, Cooney WP. Vascularized bone transfer. J Bone Joint Surg Am 1992;74:1441-1449.

[65] Arai K, Toh S, Tsubo K, Nishikawa S, Narita S, Miura H. Complications of vascularized fibula graft for reconstruction of long bones. Plast Rec Surg 2002;7:2301-6.

[66] Belt PJ, Dickinson IC, Theile DRB. Vascularised free fibular flap in bone resection and reconstruction. Br J Plast Surg 2005;58:425-30.

[67] Minami A, Kaneda K, Itoga H, Usui M. free vascularized fibular grafts. J Reconstr Microsurg 1989; 5:37-43.

[68] De Boer HH, Wood MB. Bone changes in the vascularized fibular grafts. J Bone Joint Surg Br 1989;71(3)374-378.

[69] Shpitzer T, Neligan P, Boyd B, Gullane P, Gur E, Freeman J. Leg morbidity and function following fibular free flap harvest. Ann Plast Surg 1997;38(5):460-4.

[70] Garrett A, Ducic Y, Athre RS, Motley T, Carpenter B. Evaluation of fibula free flap donor site morbidity. Am J Otolaryngol. 2006;27(1):29-32.

[71] Levin LS. Tumor reconstruction: The use of the vascularized osteoseptocutaneous fibula transplant for extremity reconstruction. Oper Tech Orthop 1998;9: 84-91.

5

Bone Grafting in Malunited Fractures

Fernando Baldy dos Reis[1] and Jean Klay Santos Machado[2]
[1]Orthopedics and Traumatology Department,
Universidade Federal de São Paulo (Unifesp), São Paulo,
[2]Porto Dias and Adventista de Belém Hospitals, Pará,
Brazil

1. Introduction

Pseudarthrosis and delayed union are two types of malunion events that can occur during fracture healing, and it is necessary to define and recognize the differences between them. Pseudarthrosis is defined as a case of consolidation failure in which a false joint is formed, including the presence of synovial fluid. Delayed union, or a delay in the fracture consolidation, is a condition where consolidation is not present and there is no evidence that it might occur, but there are no signs of movements in the focus of the lesion or of a "false joint": the bones simply do not unite (Jupiter & Rüedi, 1992; Miller & Phalen, 1947; Muller et al. 1990; Müller, 1965; Weber & Cech, 1976).

In 1986, the Food and Drug Administration (FDA) bureau defined diaphysis malunion as a situation identified at least nine months after the injury, provided the fracture shows no visible progressive signs of consolidation in the last three months. This concept applies only to diaphyses and is not a definition in cases of femoral neck or scaphoid fractures, in which the maximum periods considered for consolidation are three and four months respectively. In other cases, such as severe bone loss or active infections, the cut-off periods for a diagnosis of malunion are usually much shorter (Campbell & Boyd, 1941; Scaglietti et al. 1965; Schemitsch & Richards, 1992).

In cases of union delay, the healing process that is expected for the fracture is not interrupted; it does occur, but too slowly, unlike pseudarthrosis, in which there is an interruption in the bone healing. The process of evolution of the bone healing can be clinically and radiographically evidenced and followed up (Boyd, 1943; Ring et al. 1997).

2. Epidemiology

The incidence of malunions reported in the literature varies from 1% to 12% (Miller & Phalen, 1947, Moroni et al. 1997; Müller, 1965; Rasmussen et al. 1993) according to the severity of the primary lesion and the treatment initially used. The phenomenon is more common in men (over 80% of cases) in the third and fourth decades of life, probably due to the fact that these men are more frequently involved in risky activities (Scaglietti et al., 1965). The dominant limb is the one most affected (Weber & Cech, 1976; Wei et al. 1986; Weiland et al. 1979), probably due to intensified use of the limb in the postoperative period.

When this is associated with an inadequate surgical procedure, the risk of malunion is higher (Weber & Cech, 1976; Wei et al. 1986).

3. Etiology

Pseudarthrosis may be caused by mechanical and/or biological factors (Weber & Cech, 1976).

a. Mechanical factors involved in pseudarthrosis
-   Lack of stabilization in unstable fractures;
-   Deficient stabilization of the fracture, as in cases of fixation with plate and screws, with insufficient number of cortical elements involved in each side, fractures treated with unlocked intramedullary devices, and the use of inappropriate plates, such as the one-third tubular plate in forearm fractures
-   Fractures treated conservatively, with an insufficient immobilization period.

According to the Perren and Cordey theory (cited by Perren & Ito, 2009), osteoblasts need stability between the bone fragments in order to develop. Therefore, spaces between fragments larger than 4 mm cannot be filled by new bone tissue. In situations of high strain, the gap is filled by chondroblasts and fibroblasts, instead of bone formation cells, particularly in surgically treated cases.

b. Biological factors involved in pseudarthrosis

b1- Local:

-   Bone defects
-   Open (exposed) fractures
-   Injury to soft tissue structures close to the fractured bone, such as in direct trauma cases
-   Intensive comminution
-   Segmental fractures
-   Pathological fractures
-   Diastatic fractures
-   Soft-tissue interposition.

b2- Systemic:

-   Neuropathies
-   Diabetes mellitus
-   Malnutrition
-   Chronic smoking
-   Chronic alcoholism
-   Use of anticoagulants
-   Use of corticosteroids

4. Classification

The most commonly used classification is still the one proposed by Müller, Weber and Cech in 1976 (Weber & Cech, 1976), which divides malunited fractures into two groups: those that are vascularized and those that are avascular or unviable.

Vascularized malunions may be hypertrophic (known as "elephant's foot"), with a large callous formation, normotrophic ("horse hoof") or oligotrophic, as shown in Figure 1. Hypertrophic consolidation may be the result of mechanical problems, such as poor fixation, inadequate immobilization, and premature weight bearing on the affected limb, with reduced fractures with viable fragments. Normotrophic healing occurs after moderate fixation with plates and screws. Oligotrophic consolidation, despite being vascularized, does not present a callous formation, and occurs after an accentuated deviation, or diastasis of the fragment due to internal fixation without precise positioning of the fragments.

A   B   C

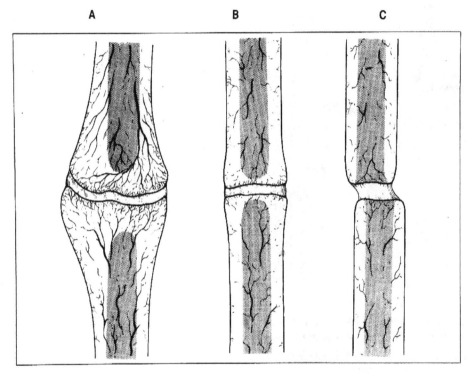

Fig. 1. Illustration of vascularized malunited fractures: "elephant's foot" (A), "horse hoof" (B) and oligotrophic (C).

Avascular malunions are classified as wedge, twisted; comminuted; by bone defects (gaps) and atrophic. As shown in Figure 2, in the case of the wedge, twisted malunion, there is an intermediate bone fragment, and the consolidation takes place only in one of the main fragments. In the case of the comminutive malunion, one or more intermediate bone fragments are necrotic, and these generally result in breaking of the plate. In consolidation failure by bone defects, there is a loss of one of the fragments. The bone extremities are viable. These cases occur after open fractures with bone loss, tumor resections or osteotomies. In the atrophic cases, osteoporotic and atrophic extremities are present, and there is an interpositioning of healing tissue, but without osteogenic potential (Weber & Cech, 1976).

A   B   C   D

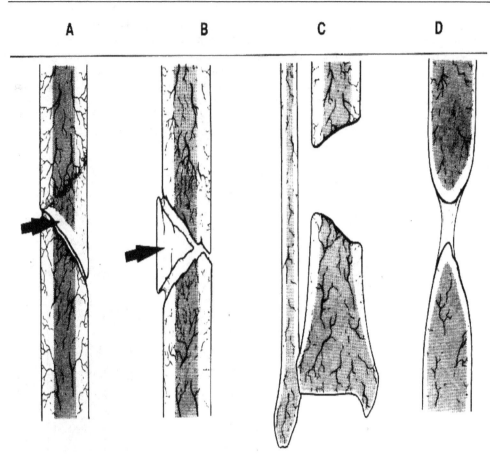

Fig. 2. Illustration of avascular malunions: wedge, twisted (A), comminutive (B), bone gap (C) and atrophic (D).

5. Signs and symptoms

Basically, patients with malunited fractures present pain when moving the limb, and when manual pressure is applied to the lesion. The presence of deformity (Figure 3) or visible mobility depends on the type of malunion (Schemitsch & Richards, 1992; Segmüller et al. 1969).

6. Imaging exams

The diagnosis of consolidation failure is, in most cases, clinical and radiographical. For the radiographic study, two incidences are enough: antero-posterior and lateral, including necessarily the satellites joints for a correct evaluation of the lesion. In situations where the diagnosis is not evident in the initial X ray, additional exams can be obtained:

- Planigraphy, in which one of the sections may show a radiotransparent line corresponding to the focus of the lesion

- Bone scintigraphy, in which the increase in captation may indicate the presence of mobility in the focus of the lesion
- Computed tomography, with 2-mm sections, which can definitely show the presence of the lesion (Figure 4).

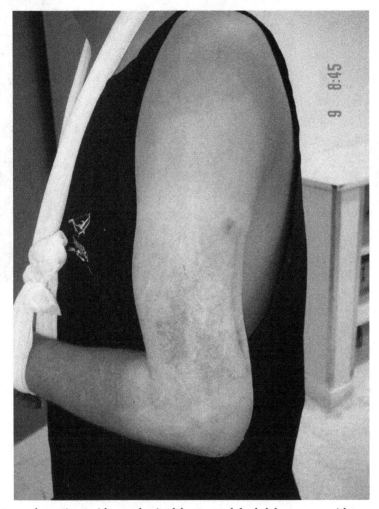

Fig. 3. Picture of a patient with a malunited fracture of the left humerus, with an evident deformity of the limb.

In patients with previous surgical treatments and in those with signs of infection, it is advisable to perform laboratory exams (blood sedimentation, c-reactive protein, complete blood count), in order to identify active infection, since latent infections do not appear in the usual laboratory exams. In imaging exams, the presence of a periosteal reaction, or signs of implant loosening, are suggestive of local infection (Barbieri et al. 1997; Muller et al. 1990; Scuderi, 1948; Spira, 1954).

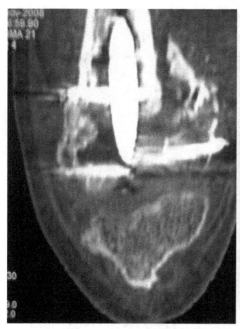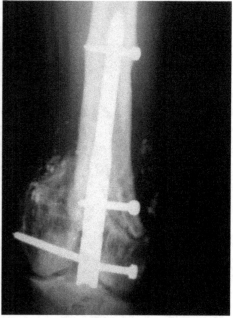

Fig. 4. Frontal section computed tomography (left) showing nonunion of the distal femur, without any evident radiographic signs (right).

7. Treatment

The treatment of malunited fractures is surgical, because the lesion results in severe anatomic and functional disorders. The method is chosen according to the type of lesion, as well as its cause: therefore, it is important to define whether the origin is mechanical or biological. In general, bone grafts are indicated in cases where the cause is either purely biological, or biological associated with a mechanical cause. Thus, vascularized and sometimes oligothophic malunited fractures have formal indication for bone grafting (dos Reis et al. 2009; Gibson & Loadman, 1948; Haddad & Drez, 1974, Nicoll, 1956).

The bone grafts used in these cases are basically (dos Reis et al. 2009; Nilsson et al. 1986; Piotrowski et al., 2005; Reis, 2001):

a. Autologous: grafted from the same patient
    1. Cancellous (spongy): used in most cases
    2. Tricortical: indicated when there is a segmental gap
    3. Segmental, which can be free or vascularized
b. Synthetic: usually made of hydroxyapatite, whether associated or not with any calcium derivative, such as tricalcium phosphate
    4. Granulated
    5. En bloc.

7.1 Surgical techniques

a.   Malunited fracture without a bone gap

Treatment consists in inserting a cancellous bone graft (best results) or synthetic, granulated graft over the lesion site. Where necessary, this may be associated with a synthesis material review (Figure 5) (Ring et al. 1997; Schemitsch & Richards, 1992; Segmüller et al. 1969; Tydings et al. 1986).

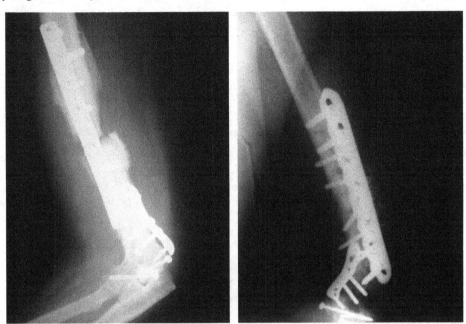

Fig. 5. Radiograph of a malunited fracture (left) of the humerus, treated with a new synthesis material and with synthetic bone grafting

b.   Malunited fracture with a partial bone gap

In this case, there are two treatment options:

b1) Using the abovementioned technique, with the bone graft filling the gap. For this, the remaining cortical bone must have viable tissue at the edges. The advantage of this method is that it preserves the bone length. The disadvantage is its dependence on the synthesis material, since the lower contact between the bone extremities requires the synthesis to be larger (Barbieri et al., 1997; dos Reis et al., 2009; Orzechowski et al., 2007; Reis, 2001).

b2) Resecting the bone extremities, in order to regularize the main fragments, followed by autologous or granulated, synthetic bone grafting. The advantage is that the procedure is less dependent on synthesis, and the disadvantage is that it shortens the bone length, which should not be less than 2 cm in the upper limbs and 5 cm in the lower limbs, to avoid functional problems (Figure 6) (Haddadr & Drez, 1974; Ilizarov, 1988; Muller et al., 1990; Müller, 1965).

c.   Malunited fracture with a segmental bone loss

In this case there are three treatment options:

c1) Treatment with an external fixation: bone transfer, especially for larger bone gaps, or in cases of acute shortening associated with lengthening outside the malunion lesion. The advantage of this method is the possibility of treating cases with infection; and the disadvantage is the morbidity associated with the technique, like pain, stiffness joint, superficial infections and many scars (Aronson, 1997; Ilizarov, 1991; Ilizarov et al., 1972; Ilizarov, 1988, Paley et al., 1989).

c2) The use of an antibiotic-impregnated cement spacer to treat the infection, over a period of six weeks. After this period, a pseudocapsule (induced membrane) is formed and used as a container for the cancellous bone graft that is inserted in the second stage. This technique was described by Masquelet and colleagues (Masquelet & Begue, 2010; Masquelet et al., 2000), and is an alternative in cases of bone loss with infection. However, its drawback is synthesis overload, since the cancellous bone graft adds little stability to the lesion site.

c3) Treatment with segmental bone graft, usually the fibula, which may be vascularized or not. This technique is indicated mainly in cases where there is major bone loss, and the graft must be included in the synthesis. Its advantage is that it preserves limb length, and its disadvantage is the complexity of the method, especially when a vascularized graft is used (Figure 7) (Miller & Phalen, 1947; Reis, 2001).

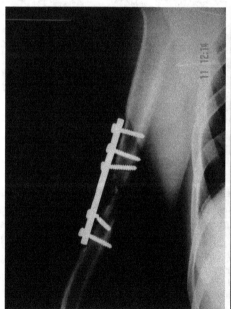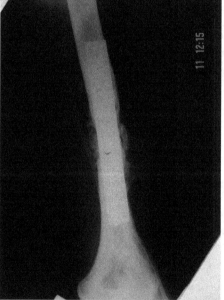

Fig. 6. Radiograph showing a nonunion of the humerus with a partial bone defect (left), treated with resection of the edges, bone shortening of 3 cm, and change of the synthesis material associated with bone grafting.

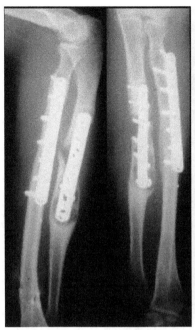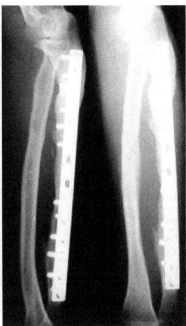

Fig. 7. Malunited ulna fracture with segmental bone loss, treated with osteosynthesis with long a dynamic compression plate (DCP) associated with bone grafting (non-vascularized fibula)

d. Special situations

d1) Malunited fracture with a bone loss in one of the forearm bones.

Because the forearm is a well-established morphofunctional unit, it is necessary to preserve compatibility of the length between the two long bones. Therefore, we may use a tricortical or a vascularized graft (mainly in gaps larger than 6 cm) in the bone that presents bone tissue loss and/or to associate this procedure with shortening of the other bone (Figure 8) (Barbieri et al., 1997; dos Reis, 2009; Reis, 2001).

d2) Nonunion with a bone loss in lower limbs

The classical indication for this kind of lesion is bone transfer with external fixation. However, particularly in cases where there are large gaps, and depending on the patient's tolerability, we usually choose the shortening-elongation method. In this case, it is left to the patient's discretion to determine whether the elongation is complete or not, but without compromising the consolidation of the malunited fracture. The lesion is submitted to compression from the start of the treatment, except in the case of bone transfer (Aronson, 1997; Ilizarov, 1991; Ilizarov et al., 1972; Ilizarov, 1988; Paley et al., 1989).

d3) Pseudoarthrosis after intramedullary nail insertion

Due to the increasingly frequent use of intramedullary nails, the occurrence of this type of nonunion has become fairly common. In these cases, the indication is usually substitution with a reamed, blocked, intramedullary nail, making the use of an autologous graft unnecessary: studies show that the effect of reaming is comparable to open cancellous bone grafting, provided the reaming is at least 2 mm larger than that of the first surgery (Figure 9) (Spira, 1954; Tydings et al., 1986).

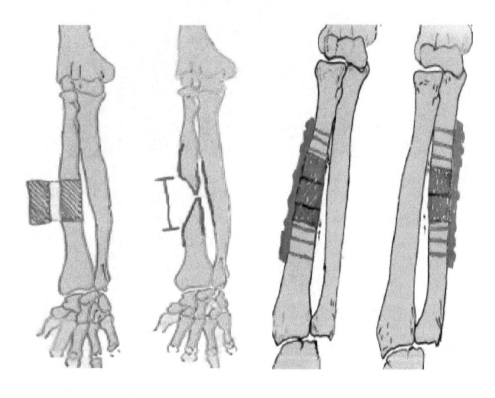

Fig. 8. Illustration showing the pre-operative surgical planning in the case of an atrophic nonunion of the radius with adjustment of the borders, grafting and ostheosynthesis with plate and screw

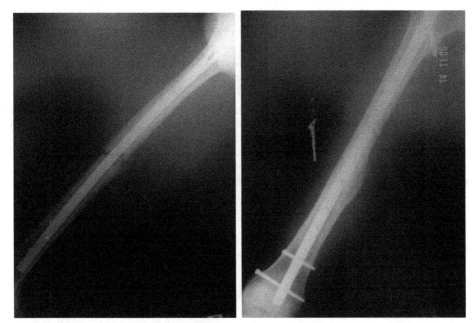

Fig. 9. Radiograph of a diaphyseal femoral nonunion (left), in a patient using a blocked intramedullary nail, treated with the substitution of the nail for a longer one with a larger caliber, resulting in consolidation (right).

8. References

Aronson, J. (1997). Limb-lengthening, skeletal reconstruction, and bone transport with the Ilizarov method. *The Journal of Bone and Joint Surgery. American Volume*, Vol.79, No.8, (August 1997), pp. 1243-58, ISSN 0021-9355.

Barbieri, CH, Mazzer, N, Aranda, CA & Pinto, MM. (1997). Use of a bone block graft from the iliac crest with rigid fixation to correct diaphyseal defects of the radius and ulna. *The Journal of Hand Surgery: Journal of the British Society for Surgery of the Hand*, Vol.22, No.3, (June 1997), pp. 395-401, ISSN 0266-7681.

Boyd, HB. (1943). The treatment of difficult and unusual non-unions. *Journal of Bone and Joint Surgery*, 25:535-52. Accessed in 2011 (May 3), Available from:
<http://www.ejbjs.org/cgi/content/abstract/25/3/535>

Campbell, WC & Boyd, HB. (1941). Fixation of onlay bone grafts by means of vitallium screws in the treatment of ununited fractures. *American Journal of Surgery*, Vol.51, (March 1941), pp. 748-56, ISSN 0002-9610.

dos Reis, FB, Faloppa, F, Fernandes, HJ, Albertoni, WM & Stahel, PF. (2009). Outcome of diaphyseal forearm fracture-nonunions treated by autologous bone grafting and compression plating. *Annals of Surgical Innovation and Research*, Vol.3, No.5, (May 2009), ISSN 1750-1164.

Gibson, A & Loadman, B. (1948). The bridging of bone defects. *The Journal of Bone and Joint Surgery. American Volume*, Vol.30A, No.2, (April 1948), pp. 381-96, ISSN 0021-9355.

Haddad, RJ Jr & Drez, D. (1974). Salvage procedures for defects in the forearm bones. *Clinical Orthopaedics and Related Research*, No.104, (October 1974), pp. 183-90, ISSN 0009-921X.

Ilizarov, GA, Kaplunov, AG, Degtiarev, VE & Lediaev, V. (1972). Lechenie lozhnykh sustavov i nesrosshikhsia perelomov, oslozhnennykh gnoinoi infektsiei, metodom kompressionno-distraktsionnogo osteosinteza [Treatment of pseudarthroses and ununited fractures, complicated by purulent infection, by the method of compression-distraction osteosynthesis]. *Ortopediia Travmatologia i Protezirovanie*, Vol.33, No.11, (November 1972), pp. 10-4, ISSN 0030-5987.

Ilizarov, GA. (1988). The principles of the Ilizarov method. *Bulletin of the Hospital for Joint Diseases Orthopaedic Institute*, Vol.48. No.1, (Spring 1988), pp. 1-11, ISSN 0883-9344.

Ilizarov, GA. (1991). Asami Group- Classification and treatment of nonunion. In: *Operative principles of Ilizarov: fracture, treatment, nonunion, osteomyelitis, lengthening deformity correction*. Bianchi-Maiocchi, A, Aronson, J, Eds, pp. 190-8, Williams & Wilkins, ISBN 978-0683007503, Baltimore.

Jupiter, JB & Rüedi, T. (1992). Intraoperative distraction in the treatment of complex nonunions of the radius. *The Journal of Hand Surgery*, Vol.17, No.3, (May 1992), pp. 416-22, ISSN 0363-5023.

Masquelet, AC & Begue, T. (2010). The concept of induced membrane for reconstruction of long bone defects. *The Orthopedic Clinics of North America*, Vol.41, No.1, (January 2010), pp. 27-37, ISSN 0030-5898.

Masquelet, AC, Fitoussi, F, Begue, T & Muller, GP. (2000). Reconstruction des os longs par membrane induite et autogreffe spongieuse [Reconstruction of the long bones by the induced membrane and spongy autograft]. *Annales de Chirurgie Plastique et Esthétique*, Vol.45, No.3, (June 2000), pp. 346-53, ISSN 0294-1260.

Miller, RC & Phalen, GS. (1947). The repair of defects of the radius with fibular bone grafts. *The Journal of Bone Joint Surgery. American volume*, Vol.29, No.3, (July 1947), pp. 629-36, ISSN 0021-9355.

Moroni, A, Rollo, G, Guzzardella, M & Zinghi, G. (1997) Surgical treatment of isolated forearm non-union with segmental bone loss. *Injury*, Vol.28, No.8, (October 1997), pp. 497-504, ISSN 0020-1383.

Muller, ME, Allgöwer, M & Shneider, R. (1991). *Manual of internal fixation of fractures*, Springer-Verlag, ISBN 4-431-52523-8, New York.

Müller, ME. (1965). Treatment of nonunions by compression. *Clinical Orthopaedics and Related Research*, Vol.43, (November-December 1965), pp. 83-92, ISSN 0009-921X.

Nicoll, EA. (1956). Treatment of gaps in long bones by cancellous insert grafts. *The Journal of Bone and Joint Surgery. British volume*, Vol.38-B, No.1, (February 1956), pp. 70-82, ISSN 0301-620X.

Nilsson, OS, Urist, MR, Dawson, EG, Schmalzried, TP & Finerman, GA. (1986). Bone repair induced by bone morphogenetic protein in ulnar defects in dogs. *The Journal of Bone and Joint Surgery. British volume*, Vol.68, No.4, (August 1986), pp. 635-42, ISSN 0301-620X.

Orzechowski W, Morasiewicz L, Dragan S, Krawczyk A, Kulej M & Mazur T (2007). Treatment of non-union of the forearm using distraction-compression osteogenesis. *Ortopedia, Traumatologia, Rehabilitacja*, Vol.9, No.4, (July-August 2007), pp. 357-65, ISSN 1509-3492.

Paley, D, Catagni, MA, Argnani, F, Villa, A, Benedetti, GB & Cattaneo, R. (1989). Ilizarov treatment of tibial nonunions with bone loss. *Clinical Orthopaedics and Related Research*, No.241, (April 1989), pp. 146-65, ISSN 0009-921X.

Perren, SM , & Ito, K. (2009). Biologia e biomecânica na consolidação óssea. In: *Princípios AO do tratamento das fraturas.* Ruedi, TP, Buckley, RE, Moran, CG, Eds. PP. 33-56, Artmed, ISBN 9788536317502, São Paulo.

Piotrowski, M, Baczkowski, B & Luczkiewicz, P. (2005). Zastosowanie litego przeszczepu korowo-gabczastego w leczeniu stawów rzekomych trzonu kosci przedramienia [Application of block of corticocancellous graft in the treatment of forearm shaft nonunions]. *Chirurgia Narzadów Ruchu i Ortopedia Polska*, Vol.70, No.1, pp. 45-7, ISSN 0009-479X.

Rasmussen, SW, Bak, K & Tøholm, C. (1993). External compression of forearm nonunion. A report on 6 cases. *Acta Orthopaedica Scandinavica*, Vol.64, No.6, (December 1993), pp. 669-70, ISSN 0001-6470.

Reis, FB. (2001). *Tratamento da pseudoartroses da diáfise dos ossos do antebraço com placa de compressão e enxertia óssea autóloga [Pseudoarthrosis treatment of the forearm shaft with compression plate and autogenous bone graft]* [Tese]. São Paulo: Universidade Federal de São Paulo. Escola Paulista de Medicina.

Ring, D, Jupiter, JB, Sanders, RA, Quintero, J, Santoro, VM, Ganz, R & Marti, RK. (1997). Complex nonunion of fractures of the femoral shaft treated by wave-plate osteosynthesis. *The Journal of Bone Joint Surgery. British volume*, Vol.79, No.2, (March 1997), pp. 289-94, ISSN 0301-620X.

Scaglietti, O, Stringa, G & Mizzau, M. (1965). Bone grafting in nonunion of the forearm. *Clinical Orthopaedics and Related Research*, Vol.43, (November-December 1965), pp. 65-76, ISSN 0009-921X.

Schemitsch, EH & Richards, RR. (1992). The effect of malunion on functional outcome after plate fixation of fractures of both bones of the forearm in adults. *The Journal of Bone and Joint Surgery. American volume*, Vol.74, No.7, (August 1992), pp. 1068-78, ISSN 0021-9355.

Scuderi, C. (1948). Restoration of long bone defects with massive bone grafts. *Journal of the American Medical Association*, Vol.137, No.13, (July 1948), pp. 1116-21, ISSN 0002-9955.

Segmüller, G, Cech, O & Bekier, A. (1969). Die osteogenese Aktivitat im Bereich der Pseudarthrose langer Röhrenknochen [Osteogenic activity in the area of pseudarthrosis of the long tubular bones]. *Zeitschrift für Orthopädie und Ihre Grenzgebiete*, Vol.106, No.3, (July 1969), pp. 599-609, ISSN 0044-3220.

Spira, E. (1954). Bridging of bone defects in the forearm with iliac graft combined with intramedullary nailing. *The Journal of Bone and Joint Surgery. British volume*, Vol.36-B, No.4, (November 1954):642-6, ISSN 0301-620X.

Tydings, JD, Martino, LJ, Kircher, M, Alfred, R & Lozman, J. (1986). The osteoinductive potential of intramedullary canal bone reamings. *Current Surgery*, Vol.43, No.2, (March-April, 1986), pp. 121-4, ISSN 0149-7944.

Weber, BG & Cech, O. (1976). *Pseudoarthrosis.* Bern, ISBN 9783456801957, Hans Huber Publishers.

Wei, FC, Chen, HC, Chuang, CC & Noordhoff, MS. (1986) Fibular osteoseptocutaneous flap: anatomic study and clinical application. *Plastic and Reconstructive Surgery*, Vol.78, No.2, (August 1986), pp. 191-200, ISSN 0032-1052.

Weiland, AJ, Kleinert, HE, Kutz, JE & Daniel, RK. (1979). Free vascularized bone grafts in surgery of the upper extremity. *The Journal of Hand Surgery*, Vol.4, No.2, (March 1979), pp. 129-44, ISSN 0363-5023.

Part 4

Orthopaedic Surgery

6

Osteonecrosis Femoral Head Treatment by Core Decompression and ILIAC CREST-TFL Muscle Pedicle Grafting

Sudhir Babhulkar

Indira Gandhi Medical College, Nagpur,
Sushrut Hosp, Research Centre & PGI, Nagpur,
India

1. Introduction

Osteonecrosis of femoral head is a painful disabling condition seen in association with many disorders like corticosteroids consumption, alcohol abuse, haemoglobinopathy (sickle cell disease, coagulopathies), certain renal, hepatic and skin disorders commonly affecting young patients ranging from 20-40 years.[1-3] It is now recognized as a major musculo-skeletal problem mostly affecting the young people in their productive years of life. It is often characterized by relentless progression despite treatment, resulting in to subchondral fracture, collapse and painful arthrosis.[4] Hence it is essential to diagnose and treat the patients of osteonecrosis early to prevent any further disintegration and collapse of femoral head. Advanced osteonecrosis with secondary osteoarthritis is reported in 5% to 18% of total patients undergoing total hip replacement in the US.[4-7] Aim of the treatment in osteonecrosis is to reduce the intraosseous pressure and to perform the head-preserving procedure, which will cause early revascularization of ischemic head. Various types of muscle pedicle grafting after core decompression are indicated early in the disease, depending upon the stage of the disease and have shown excellent results in revascularization of femoral head and prevention of collapse.

Once diagnosed it is desirable to subject the patient to early surgical intervention. Rationale for the treatment of osteonecrosis of femoral head requires a lot of consideration. Of prime importance is the age of patients. Whether both hips are affected, etiology of the associated diseases, demands and requirement of the patients, and the stage of the disease when the patient presents for treatment are equally important. The treatment is planned according to ARCO's classification[8] & Steinberg staging[9]. Only core decompression may relieve the pain but it does not achieve revascularization of femoral head. Hence core decompression should always be supplemented by one of the procedures of bone grafting. To achieve early vascularisation, vascular pedicle grafting using deep circumflex iliac vessel with iliac crest is a very useful, but preoperative femoral angiography is mandatory to confirm the presence of deep circumflex iliac artery pedicle[10]. This procedure is technically demanding, tedious and time consuming and may not be feasible bilaterally in one sitting. However Muscle pedicle graft using tensor fascia lata graft is very easy and is commonly performed whenever both hips need simultaneous surgery in one sitting. In the past, muscle pedicle graft using quadratus femoris (Meyer's procedure) [11] was propagated in the treatment of osteonecrosis, but it did not achieve satisfactory early revascularization and came in disrepute since the results were not encouraging. Dr DP Baksi[12] reported treatment of osteonecrosis by multiple drilling and muscle pedicle grafting by use of TFL graft with relief of pain and improvement in the hip movements. Though vascularised pedicle graft by using part of iliac crest with deep circumflex iliac vessels is more advantageous since high percentage of marrow and osteogenic cells survive within a living graft, it is difficult to perform this surgery on both hips in one sitting. As per our Institutional philosophy we prefer to operate both hips in the same sitting since it reduces the hospital stay, the cost of drugs and many cases patient may not turn up for surgery on the opposite hip, especially the poor compliance group of patients. Hence use of Muscle pedicle graft of tensor fascia lata along with iliac crest after core decompression is commonly advocated when bilateral hips are involved and surgery is recommended early in single sitting.

Finding	0	1	2	3	4
Finding	All present techniques normal or non diagnostic	X-ray and CT are normal. At least ONE of the below is positive	NO CRESCENT SIGN: X-RAY ABNORMAL: Sclerosis, lysis, focal porosis	Crescent Sign on the X-ray and/ or flattening of articular surface of femoral head	OSTEOARTHRITIS joint space narrowing, acetabular changes, joint destruction
Finding	X-ray, CT, Scintigraph, MRI	Scintigraph, MRI,Quantitate on MRI	X-ray, CT, Scintigraph MRI, QUANTITATE MRI & X-ray	X-ray, CT only * Quantitate on X-ray	X-ray only
Finding	NO	Medial	Central Lateral		NO
Finding	NO	QUANTITATION % Area Involvement Minimal A<15% Moderate B 15-30% Extensive C>30%	Length of crescent A < 2mm B 2-4 mm C >4 mm	% surface collapse dome depression A< 15% B – 15-30% C> 30%	NO

Table 1. ARCO Classification

The natural history of osteonecrosis of femoral head, before the development of crescent sign or before the collapse of the femoral head, has never been well defined. The possibility of progression to collapse is thought to increase after the development of an abnormality that can be seen on plainradiograph and the course of collapse may be highly variable and unknown[7]. It is generally agreed that symptomatic radiographically abnormal hip will progress to collapse of the femoral head when treated nonoperatively[7].To avoid these complications and to avoid early replacement arthroplasty in young patients many operative procedures to salvage the femoral head are in vogue. Head preserving operation of core decompression and various types of bone grafting certainly gave excellent results in early stage of osteonecrosis. Despite the many reports on the utility of various operative procedures no single method has uniformly demonstrated the arrest of the disease or prevention of collapse of the femoral head effectively. Core decompression only gave good clinical results initially(Ficat & Arlet)[13, 14,] but the long term results were poor.[11] The use of nonvascularised tibial (Phemister) or fibular bone graft (Boettcher & Bonfiglio)[15] is useful only in the early stages but in later stages, the results were very poor. Subarticular curettage and cancellous bone grafting failed to relieve pain and prevent progressive collapse of the femoral head.[16,17] Meyers[11] reported use of fresh cancellous graft combined with Quadratus femoris muscle pedicle graft which gave good results in stage I & II, but was unsatisfactory in stage III & IV. Though pain and deformity improved initially, vascularisation of femoral head was poor.

The vascularized fibular grafting is associated with better clinical and radiographic results than is nonvascularized fibular grafting in precollapse hips[7]. However, the successful use of free vascularized bone grafts requires a meticulous process of procuring the vascular fibula with microanastomosis to the recipient site. The microsurgical procedures require specialized training equipment and expertise.

The TFL muscle pedicle graft by using part of iliac crest described in this article is easy to perform and does not require any special equipment or technique, and still has the advantages of increased vascularity like vascularised bone graft (Fig 1A-1H). We analyzed and report a series of patients of osteonecrosis of femoral head treated by core decompression and TFL muscle pedicle graft of part of iliac crest.

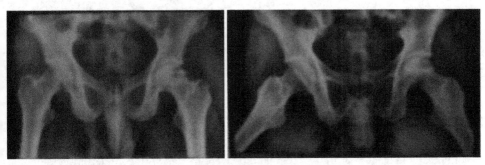

LD – 52 years male Steroid Induced ON femoral head left side

Fig. 1. 1A, 1B– Pre op X-ray 52 year's male Steroid Induced ON femoral head left side

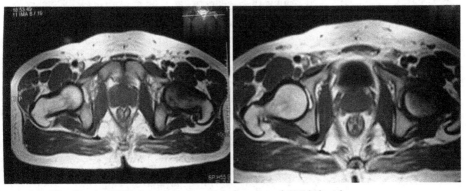

Fig. 1. 1C, 1D – Pre op MRI showing classical changes of ON left side

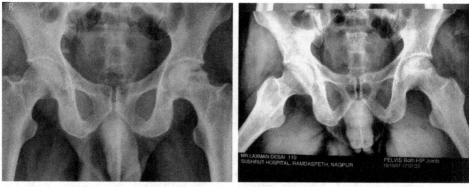

Fig. 1. 1E, 1F – Immediate Post op X ray after CD & TFL draft

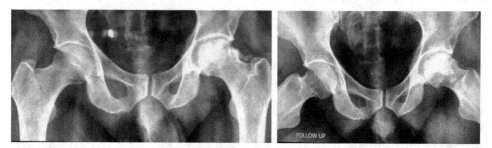

Fig. 1. 1G, 1H – Post op 3 years follow up X ray after CD & TFL draft showing good revascularization and restoration of contour of femoral head left side

2. Material & methods

This article reports the study of 68 patients of osteonecrosis femoral head, affecting 92 femoral heads in stage II & III, wherein 90 hips were treated with core decompression and Iliac crest-TFL muscle pedicle grafting by using part of iliac crest with Tensor Fascia lata (TFL) pedicle in a duration of 16 years, from Jan.95 to Dec.2010 with a minimum follow up for three years. All patients were young 16-52 years of age with a mean age of 30 years.

Forty four patients had unilateral affection where as twenty four patients had bilateral involvement, but on twenty two occasions bilateral TFL grafting was done in one sitting, whereas two patients in bilateral group were operated by TFL muscle pedicle graft on one side & free fibular grafting on the opposite side in single sitting (Fig 2A-2H, Fig 3A-3G). Thus TFL Grafting procedure was performed on total 90 hips in 68 patients. At our Institute many patients of Sickle cell disease with osteonecrosis are studied and treated, where the procedure of vascular pedicle grafting is not performed on any patient, because of the possibility of high prevalence of thrombosis in the vascular pedicle in this disease. Similarly in patients with bilateral involvement, surgery of TFL grafting in one sitting is preferred to vascular pedicle grafting, mainly because of the long time required for vascular pedicle procedure. Amongst 68 patients, 28 patients (42%) were following Alcohol abuse, 21 patients (30%) were following consumption of corticosteroids & 19 patients had sickle cell haemoglobinopathy (28%). The demography of patients is shown in the Chart 2. Amongst

24 Bilateral hips, 17 patients had stage III on one side & stage II on other side. Wherein 7 patients had stage III in both hips.

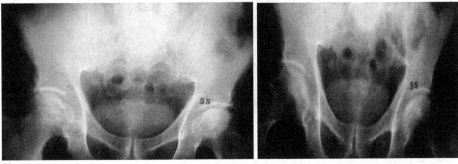

SCS

Fig. 2. 2A, 2B – Pre op X-ray 50 years male Steroid Induced ON femoral head both sides

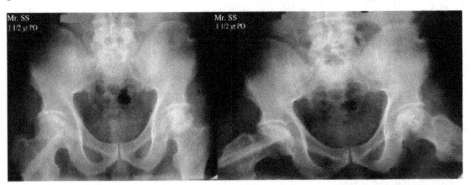

Fig. 2. 2C, 2D – Post op 1.5 years follow up X ray after CD & TFL graft on left side & free fibular graft on right side showing good revascularization and restoration of contour of femoral head

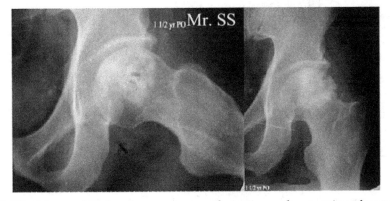

Fig. 2. 2E, 2F – 1.5 years PO showing good revascularization and restoration of contour of femoral head on left side after CD & TFL graft

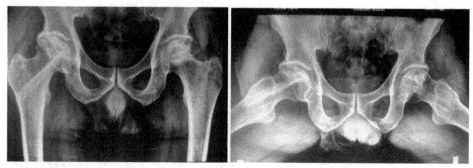

Fig. 2. 2G, 2H – 9 years PO showing good revascularization and restoration of contour of femoral head on left side after CD & TFL graft with good hip joint space.

Stage of Disease	Number of Hips	Male Hips	Female Hips	Age of the patient			
				16-20	21-30	31-40	41 & Above
Stage II A B C	33 - 15 18	20	13	2	11	16	4
Stage III A B C	57 6 36 15	36	21	4	18	22	13

Table 2. Showing demography of patients affecting 90 Hips operated by TFL grafting showing stages, age & Sex.

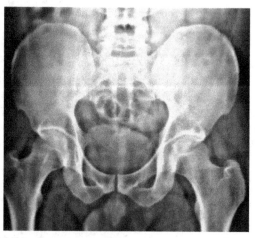

RC 28 year male Alcohol Induced

Fig. 3. 3A – X ray showing Alcohol induced ON both sides in 31 years male

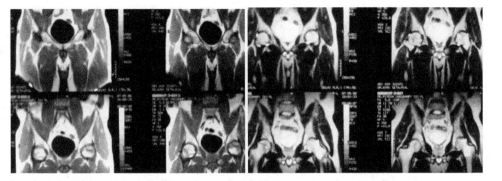

Fig. 3. 3B, 3C – MRI showing bilateral ON femoral heads

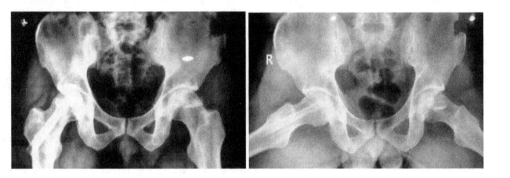

Fig. 3. 3D, 3E – 12 weeks PO after CD & TFL graft left side & free fibular graft right side

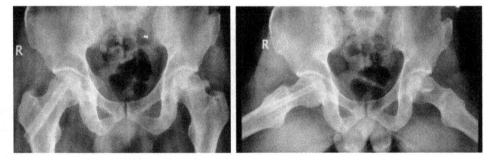

Fig. 3. 3F, 3G – 1 year PO after CD & TFL graft left side & free fibular graft right side showing good consolidation of TFL graft left side with restoration of normal femoral head contour

2.1 Operative technique

Patient after spinal anesthesia, is put in supine position with the sandbag underneath the gluteal region on the operative side. A curvilinear incision is taken on lateral side of hip extending from the iliac crest about 5 cm posterior to Anterior superior iliac spine and to the greater trochanter and extending downwards about 2 cm below the base of greater trochanter in the subtrochanteric region. The iliac crest should be exposed, freed from inner lip by erasing three abdominal muscles till you just reach about 2 cm. Similarly the iliac crest with attached tensor fascia lata on external surface should be exposed. The cleavage between Sartorius and tensor fascia lata is identified. An incision is made between anterior & middle fibers of TFL and clearly 2 - 3 cm width of TFL middle fibers are separated up to the iliac crest. With pneumatic saw osteotomy of iliac crest is done superiorly, and about 2 - 3 cm distally and medially with isolation of TFL graft externally. This isolated iliac crest graft with TFL pedicle is best done by subperiosteal separation of muscles on either side of lip of the ilium without disturbing the vascular supply. The desired size of TFL with full width of iliac crest is raised & retracted downwards with attached fibers of TFL. The TFL muscle pedicle graft just prepared gets its vascular supply from the superior gluteal artery and ascending branch of lateral circumflex femoral artery. The reflected pedicle of TFL with fibers of gluteus minimus muscle is erased from the outer surface of ilium and is retracted downwards and brought down up to the anterior capsule of the involved hip joint. The hip capsule is opened with T shaped incision. The anterior capsule and thickened synovium is excised. The ischemic necrotic segment is exposed and examined for its deformation & change in the contour. A small window is made anteriorly at the junction of articular surface of the femoral head and anterior surface of the neck of the femur by pneumatic drill. Under image intensifier through this window, serial reaming is done in the ischemic segment of the femoral head right up to the subchondral region in all the directions. Care is taken not to perforate the articular surface. Subsequently the entire necrotic tissue is removed by curette which creates a big void in the head of the femur usually in the upper quadrant of the femoral head, wherein inferior quadrant is usually not disturbed. With the special instrument & punch-impactor the deformed femoral head with articular cartilage is raised superiorly to match its original shape under IITV in all the direction. The created void is partially filled and packed with little cancellous bone removed from the iliac crest after performing the osteotomy. Subsequently the retracted & raised pedicle of TFL with iliac crest is prepared nicely to repose through the window defect at the head neck junction. Two holes are made superiorly & inferiorly in the femoral neck by of 2 mm drill bits. Similarly the two holes are prepared in the pedicle of iliac bone with TFL graft. Subsequently the TFL pedicle is impacted in to the head under image control right up to the subchondral region of femoral neck and the graft tied by No.1 Vickryl to the femoral neck. Additionally, the muscle belly is also stitched to the capsule inferiorly & superiorly. The suction drain is kept at the hip & iliac crest site and wound is closed in layers. In bilateral cases, the similar procedure is performed in the same sitting on the opposite side.

2.2 Post operative protocol

Postoperatively the limb-Hip is kept in 20-degree abduction and 30 degree flexion and 10 degree of internal rotation to avoid tension on the vascular pedicle. The patient is mobilized after 15 days in bed and after 4-6 weeks patient can be mobilized out of bed on non-weight bearing crutch walking if only one hip is operated. Whereas in bilateral cases, the patient is advised bed rest with mobilsation of hips after 4 weeks and weight bearing started after 10 weeks only. The patient is allowed partial weight bearing after 10 weeks and full weight bearing after 14-16 weeks.

2.3 Follow-up

Follow-up by clinical and radiological examination was done every 3 months for one year, every six months for next five years and then yearly follow up thereafter. Harris hip score system was used for assessment of the results. The follow up period varied from three to sixteen years. Post operatively Bone scan & Digital subtraction arteriogram was done in twenty patients comprising of ten each in stage II & III, at the end of 12 weeks, which showed hundred percent of patency and viability of the TFL muscle pedicle graft.

2.4 Results

The patients had good clinical improvement with relief from pain and improvement in the range of movements. The radiological improvement was judged by diminishen of density and attempt at revascularization as seen by healing of cystic changes, disappearance of crescent sign and restoration of normal trabecular pattern and shape of femoral head. Almost all patients had good relief from pain with good improvement in the range of movements. As per Harris Hip score results, there was improvement in the score of > 25 points in 70 % cases while in fifty % had improvement in the score of more than 28 points in both the stages. The mean +SD improvement in Harris Hip score at 3 year's follow up was 27.6 + 6.4. The difference in the preoperative and postoperative score across the whole sample was significant ($P < 0.05$)

Stage II: Seventy percent of stage II hips completely improved without any deterioration and had complete relief from pain. No patient progressed to stage III postoperatively.

Stage III: About 20% patients of stage III had residual low intensity pain for about 30 weeks. About 30% patients had painless limp for 24-30 weeks with restriction of flexion beyond 100 Degrees. Eight percent patient (5 patients) progressed to further collapse, got deformed but without any progression to arthrosis. Out of this, in four percent patients (3 patients) surgery of total hip joint was advised.

3. Discussion

Need to treat ischemia of femoral head is becoming more common since many cases are detected in early stages in young patients. One must consider the possibility of osteonecrosis if individual has pain in the vicinity of hip, that had history of chronic alcoholism, corticosteroid consumption, associated disease like sickle cell disease, Gauchers, Gout etc[18-21]. Early diagnosis prior to the appearance of radiological changes is crucial in the treatment of ischemic necrosis. Its diagnosis is based on clinical examination and by bone scan, CT, and MRI, as osteonecrosis is the response to the vascular impairment of the bone marrow circulation. X-ray examination is of limited value in early stage, but has importance in staging since it helps in planning the treatment and the prognosis. The X-ray become positive late in the condition after the process of repair has started. The ischemic death of bony and marrow tissues occur in osteonecrosis. Different imaging modalities provide different information on the mineralized and non-mineralized component of the bone. Though bone scan is also important, MRI has dramatically improved the diagnosis of osteonecrosis, and in about 30-70% cases of femoral head osteonecrosis, the other hip is affected in due course of time[18, 22]. Hence, it is necessary to rule out early involvement of the contralateral hip, which is asymptomatic by either bone scan or MRI. MRI is the most accurate imaging modality for the diagnosis of osteonecrosis of femoral head, especially in the early stages when there are only bone marrow changes[23]. Characteristic MRI signal alterations in the anterosuperior portion of the femoral head surrounded by a band of low signal intensity on T1- and T2-weighted images represent the diagnostic criteria of osteonecrosis[25-27]. The occurrence of a double-line sign on the T2-weighted image represents a pathognomonic sign, but its absence does not rule out the diagnosis of osteonecrosis. Marcus et al., Steinberg et al., Ficat and Arlet, and ARCOs classification[28,7,8-29] are the various staging systems in vogue for diagnosis of osteonecrosis, but with inherent problems of low reliability. The Association Research Circulation Osseous (ARCO) has proposed a new international classification system including radiographs, computed tomography (CT), bone scans, and MRI[8]. This classification system incorporates the lesion size and the lesion location. Quantitation (% area involvement of femoral head, length of crescent sign, % surface collapse, and dome depression) and location of the lesion (medial, central or lateral) represent important prognostic factors. This ARCOs classification has been proposed as the preferred system for the future, which is used in this study.

Core decompression offers the opportunity to study histological changes of early bone ischemia. It also achieves reduction in the symptoms of pre-collapse stage of ischemic necrosis because of reduction of pressure in the compartment. Barring exceptional circumstances, there is hardly any role of conservative treatment of osteonecrosis of femoral head and surgery is rendered inevitable.

Steinberg et al. reported that progression occurred in 92% of 48 hips that had undergone nonoperative management[30,31]. While observing the patients with protected weight bearing, more than 85% patients had collapse of femoral head at 2 years when symptomatic hips with stage I and II were left untreated. Many studies have shown that nonoperative treatment yields poor results. The only condition for which the protected weight bearing might be effective is a type A lesion i.e. involvement of medial aspect of femoral head. No drugs have been useful and specific in the treatment of osteonecrosis, though recently the use of Alendronate has been advised. Once diagnosed, it is desirable to subject the patient to early surgical intervention. Rationale for the treatment of osteonecrosis of femoral head requires a lot of consideration. Prime consideration should be given to the age of the patient, whether both hips are affected, etiology of the associated diseases, functional demands of the patients, and the stage of the disease when the patient presents for treatment. Only core decompression may relieve the pain but is not useful for revascularization of femoral head; hence, core decompression should always be supplemented by one of the procedures of bone grafting. Core decompression is an effective treatment in the pre-radiological and precollapse stage of avascular necrosis of the femoral head, [18, 32, 33] especially if coupled with bone grafting. Jones analyzed nine studies and showed that in 218 of 369 patients (59%), where core decompression was performed in the precollapse stage, failed to prevent the progressive collapse[34-36]. Steinberg et al[19,30,31] concluded that core decompression provided more predictable pain relief and changed the indications for arthroplasty more consistently than conservative management. However, only core decompression should be avoided, and it must be coupled with bone grafting in the tract of core to avoid iatrogenic fractures.[10, 37] Despite many reports on salvage procedure, no method has clearly demonstrated the arrest of disease before subchondral fracture or slow down of the progression of collapse of femoral head and arthrosis. The use of a nonvascularized bone graft, as originally described by Phemister, has had variable success in the treatment of osteonecrosis. Marcus et al[28] reported satisfactory clinical results in seven out of eleven hips at the time of short-term follow up (range: 24 years). The other workers concluded that Phemister bone-grafting technique is not effective once collapse has occurred. Boettcher etal.[15] reported success in 27 (71%) of 38 hips 6 years after nonvascularized tibial strut grafting. However, a longer-term evaluation (performed at a mean of 14 years postoperatively) that included the original 38 hips in the study by Boettcher et al. found that only 16 (29%) of 56 hips still had a good result.[38] Once the crescent sign appears without collapse, it is desirable to couple the bone grafting procedure in addition to the core decompression, preferably vascular or muscle pedicle grafting, to achieve early revascularization.[39, 10, 12.]

Vascularized pedicle graft by using part of iliac crest with deep circumflex iliac vessels is more advantageous since high percentage of marrow and osteogenic cells survive within a living graft, which helps for early vascularization[10, 40-44]. However, muscle pedicle graft using tensor fascia lata graft is very easy and is commonly performed whenever both hips need simultaneous surgery. Muscle pedicle graft using quadratus femoris (Meyers procedure) [11] was also propagated in the treatment of osteonecrosis, but it did not achieve satisfactory early revascularization and went into disrepute since the results were not encouraging, though Meyers reported the success rate of 57% and Baksi[12] reported 93% good results. Use of tensor fascia lata graft is commonly advocated when bilateral hips are involved and surgery is performed in the single sitting. The study by Plakseychuk et al[42, 43] on free vascular fibular grafting showed better clinical results and prevention of radiographic signs of progression and collapse of the femoral head more frequently than does nonvascularized fibular grafting. A marked difference with regard to signs of radiographic progression and collapse was noted between the A and B subgroups in the precollapse groups (Stages I, and II). The potential disadvantages of vascularized fibular grafting are a longer operation time, need of microvascular technique, leaves a longer operative scar, and is associated with more donor site morbidity such as ankle instability, toe-clawing, subtrochanteric fracture, and heterotopic ossification. To achieve early vascularization TFL muscle pedicle grafting along with iliac crest is very useful. This procedure is easy and is technically not demanding.

The TFL grafting provides a significant benefit for hips in Stages II and III. The rationale of this procedure (Fig 4A-4F, Fig 5A-5E) of TFL pedicle bone grafting is based on the following three points:

1. Decompression of the femoral head, which acts as compartment syndrome following increased intraosseous pressure and interrupts the circulation that is thought to contribute to the disease
2. Excision of the necrotic tissue, which inhibits revascularization of the head
3. Filling of the defect that is created after core and filled with TFL muscle pedicle with iliac crest, acts, an osteoinductive cancellous graft, which is viable and supports the subchondral surface and enhances the revascularization process.

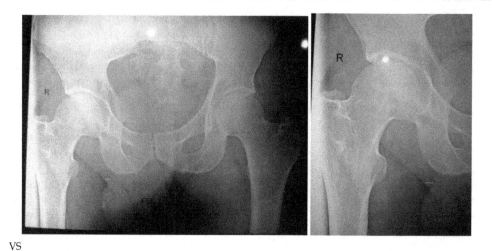

VS

Fig. 4. 4A, 4B – X ray showing Alcohol induced ON right side in 36 years male

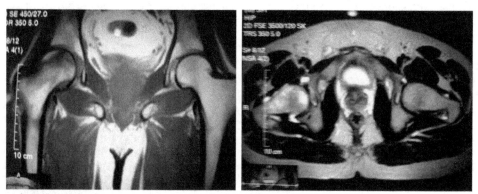

Fig. 4. 4C, 4D – MRI showing ON femoral head right side

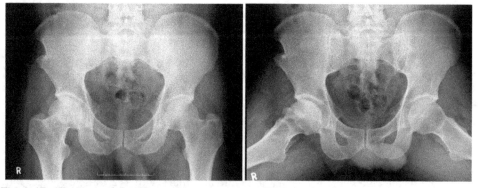

Fig. 4. 4E, 4F – X ray showing good incorporation of TFL graft maintenance of articular surface of femoral head at the end of 2 years follow up

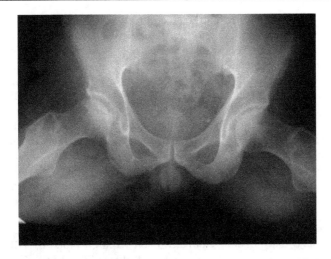

TH

Fig. 5. 5A – X ray showing Alcohol induced ON both sides in 45 years male

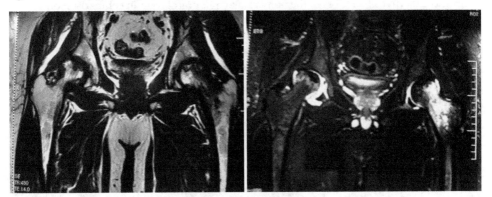

Fig. 5. 5B, 5C – MRI showing classical changes of AVN both femoral heads

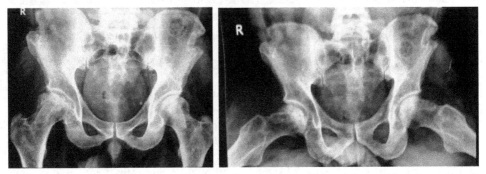

Fig. 5. 5D, 5E – 12 months PO CD & TFL graft in one sitting showing good incorporation of graft and showing good restoration of articular surface

It does not require advanced training of microsurgical technique nor any special equipment and can be performed by any average orthopaedic surgeon. Morbidity of the donor site is minimal and operative time required is comparable to total hip arthroplasty, and all problems and obstacles associated with vascularized fibular graft are avoided by this technique. Head-preserving operation of core decompression and TFL pedicle grafting certainly gives excellent results in stages II and III. The prognosis of stages II and III is fairly good, whereas in stage IV, it is not satisfactory since about 1/3 of the stage IV group are likely to progress further and may require total hip joint replacement or resurfacing operations. Prosthetic replacement is frequently an unappealing option for patients who have osteonecrosis because many patients are young and the etiological factors associated with the disease are also associated with complications after total hip arthroplasty, hemiarthroplasty, and surface replacement. At our institute, many patients of sickle cell disease with osteonecrosis are studied and treated, by this procedure of TFL Muscle pedicle grafting. Out of 103 patients treated by Urbanaiak et al[6] by free vascular fibular grafting, total hip replacement was performed in 34% cases in stages II and III within 5 years. There was survivorship and the probability of conversion within 5 years to THR rate of 11% in stage II and 23% survival for stage III. In the study of Shin Yoon Kim, [38] the rate of conversion to total hip replacement was 13% (three of 23 hips) in the vascularized graft group and 22% (five of 23 hips) in the nonvascularized graft group in comparison only three patients out of 68 of TFL muscle pedicle grafting was advised total hip replacement in the present series at the end of 16 years (Fig 6A-6F). The hips treated with TFL muscle pedicle

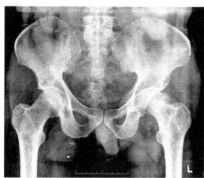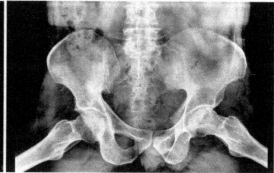

SR - 52 years

Fig. 6. 6A, 6B – X ray showing Alcohol induced ON femoral heads both sides Stage II – Right side, & Stage – III left side in 52 years male

grafting seemed to have less dome depression of the femoral head and the retention of sphericity, probably because of more rapid revascularization and increased osteoinductive potential of the pedicle graft. It has been observed that there is an early failure of total hip replacement in osteonecrosis than in age-matched patients with other diagnosis because of abnormal remodeling of bones and subsidence of prosthesis because of poor quality of proximal femoral bone[42]. Other contributory factors for failure are ongoing systemic disease, defects in mineral metabolism, use of steroids, and high level of activity in young patients and increased body weight. Hence, we prefer to delay or eliminate the need for hip replacement by performing head-preserving surgeries[10, 37], of which core decompression and TFL muscle pedicle grafting are a choice of surgery, especially in bilateral cases and patients with Sickle cell disease with stage II and III. Out of 68 patients, only five patients progressed to collapse, and surgery of joint replacement was advised in three patients.

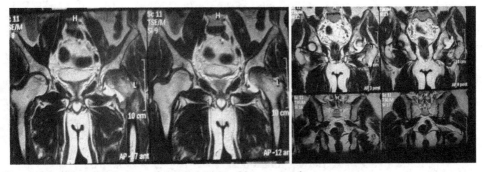

Fig. 6. 6C, 6D – MRI showing bilateral ON in 52 years male

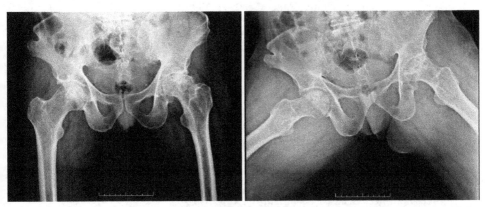

Fig. 6. 6E, 6F – PO 1 year X ray showing collapse of femoral head with arthritic changes left side, good incorporation of graft right side with good joint space. Patient is advised THA left side

4. Conclusion

Basically osteonecrosis of femoral head is a multifactorial, heterogeneous group of disorder that leads to final common pathology of mechanical failure of femoral head. In this study more than seventy percent patients had osteonecrosis because of alcohol abuse (42%) & steroid consumption (30%) and in 28 percent cases belonged to Sickle cell disease. It is common in young age group where conservative surgical approach is chosen, than a radical approach of reconstructive surgery. If diagnosed early head preserving operation of core decompression and TFL Muscle pedicle bone grafting yields excellent result. Essentially the result depends on the preoperative condition of the joint and the site of necrotic focus and the associated disease, which may be the cause of osteonecrosis. From our experience, if the ischemic necrosis of femoral head is diagnosed early in stage II, & III core decompression and TFL Muscle pedicle grafting gives very good results. In stage III, even if there is slight collapse with deformation, the depressed segment can be elevated and deformity corrected after elevation and bone grafting. Out of 68 patients with 90 hips only five patients progressed to collapse and surgery of joint replacement was advised in three patients of stage III. The long standing effect of surgery were excellent with great improvement in the Harris hip score, achieving improvement in the score between 70-80 points in majority of patients at the final follow up period.

5. References

[1] Glimcher MJ, Kenzora JE: The biology of osteonecrosis of the human femoral head and its clinical implications: Part III. Discussion of the etiology and genesis of the pathological sequelae; comments on treatment. *Clin Orthop* 1979; 140:273-312.

[2] Herndon JH, Aufranc OE: Avascular necrosis of the femoral heaad in the adult. A review of its incidence ina variety of conditions. *Clin Orthop* 1972; 86:43-62.

[3] Glimcher MJ, Kenzora JE: The biology of osteonecrosis of the human femoral head and its clinical implications: Part II. The pathological changes in the femoral head as an organ and in the hip joint. *Clin Orthop* 1979; 139:283-312.

[4] Kenzora JE, Glimcher MJ: Pathogenesis of idiopathic osteonecrosis: The ubiquitous crescent sign. *Orthop Clin North Am* 1985; 16:681-696.

[5] Mankin HJ: Nontraumatic necrosis of bone (osteonecrosis). *N Eng J Med* 1992; 326:1473-1479.

[6] Mont MA, Hungerford DS: Non-traumatic avascular necrosis of the femoral head. *J Bone Joint Surg* 1995; 77A: 459-474.

[7] Urbaniak JR, Coogan PG, Gunneson EB, et al: Treatment of osteonecrosis of the femoral head with free vascularised fibular grafting: A long term follow up study of one hundred and three hips. *J Bone Joint Surg* 1995; 77A: 681-694.

[8] Gardeniers JWM: ARCO international classification of osteonecrosis. *ARCO News 1993;* 5:79-82.

[9] Steinberg ME, Hayken GD, and Steinberg DR: A quantitative system for staging avascular necrosis. *J Bone Joint Surg* 1995; 77B: 34-41.

[10] Babhulkar SS: Osteonecrosis of femoral head: Treatment by core decompression and vascular pedicle grafting IJO – Vol 43 January Issue 1, March 2009: 27-35

[11] Meyers MH. The treatment of osteonecrosis of the hip with fresh osteochondral allografts and with the muscle-pediclegraft technique. *Clini Orthop* 1978; 130: 202-209.

[12] Baksi DP. Treatment of osteonecrosis of the femoral head by drilling and muscle-pedicle bone grafting. *J Bone Joint Surg* (Br) *1991; 73-B: 241-245.*

[13] Ficat P, Arlet J, Hungerford DS (eds): *Ischaemia and Necrosis of Bone.* Baltimore, MD, Williams & Wilkins, 1980.

[14] Ficat RP: Idiopathic bone necrosis of the femoral head: Early diagnosis and treatment. *J Bone Joint Surg* 1985; 67B: 3-9.

[15] Boettcher WG, Bonfigilo M, Smith K: Non-traumatic necrosis of the femoral head: II. Experiences in treatment. *J Bone Joint Surg* 1970; 52A: 322-329.

[16] Steinberg ME, Brighton CT, Hayken GD et al. Electrical stimulation in the treatment of Osteonecrosis of the femoral head – a 1 year follow-up. *Orthop. Clin North Am* 1985; 16: 747-756.

[17] Steinberg ME, Hayken GD, Steinberg DR. The conservative management of avascular necrosis of the femoral head. In Bone Circulation. Edited by Arlet A, Ficat RP, Hungerford DS. Baltimore; Williams and Wilkins. 1984: 334-337.

[18] Hungerford DS, Jones LC: Diagnosis of osteonecrosis of the femoral head. In Schoutens A, Arlet J , Gardeniers JWM, et al (eds): Bone Circulation and Vascularisation in Normal and Pathological Conditions. New York, NY, Plenum Press, *1993,pp 265-275*

[19] Steinberg ME, Hayken GD, and Steinberg DR: A quantitative system for staging avascular necrosis. *J Bone Joint Surg* 1995; 77B: 34-41.

[20] Arlet J, Ficat P: Forage-biopsie de la tete femorale dans l'osteonecrose primitive. Observations histo-pathologiques portant sur huit forgaes. Rev Rhumat *1964; 31:257-264.*

[21] Bradway JK, Morrey BF: The natural history of the silent hip in bilateral atraumatic osteonecrosis. *J Arthroplasty* 1993; 8:383-387.

[22] Mitchell DG, Steinberg ME, Dalinka MK et al: Magnetic resonance imaging of the ischaemic hip: Alterations within the osteonecrotic , viable, and reactive zone. *Clin Orthop* 1989; 244:60-77

[23] Shimizu K, Moriya H, Akita T et al: Prediction of collapse with magnetic resonance imaging of avascular necrosis of the femoral head. *J Bone Joint Surg* 1994; 76A:215-223.

[24] Beltran J, Knight CT, Zuelzer WA et al: Core decompression for avascular necrosis of the femoral head: Correlation between long-term results and preoperative MR staging. *Radiology* 1990; 175:533-536.

[25] Robinson HJ Jr: Success of core decompression in the management of early stages of avascular necrosis: A four-year prospective study. Proceedings of the American Academy of Orthopaedic Surgeons 59th Annual Meeting, Washington DC, Park Ridge, IL, *American Academy of Orthopaedic Surgeons*, 1992, p177.

[26] Norman A, Bullough P: The radiolucent crescent line: An early diagnostic sign of avascular necrosis of the femoral head. *Bull Hosp Joint Dis* 1963; 24:99-104

[27] Harris WH Tarumatic arthritis of the hip, J Bone Joint Surg(Am) 1969; 51A:738-743.

[28] Marcus ND, Enneking WF, Massam RA. The silent hip in idiopathic aseptic necrosis: treatment by bone grafting. *J Bone Joint Surg (Am)* 1973; 55-A: 1351-66.

[29] Kerboul M, Thomine J, Postel M et al: The conservative surgical treatment of idiopathic aseptic necrosis of the femoral head. *J Bone Joint Surg* 1974; 56B: 291-296.

[30] Steinberg ME, Brighton CT, Hayken GD et al. Electrical stimulation in the treatment of Osteonecrosis of the femoral head – a 1 year follow-up. *Orthop. Clin North Am* 1985; 16: 747-756.

[31] Steinberg ME, Hayken GD, Steinberg DR. The conservative management of avascular necrosis of the femoral head. In Bone Circulation. Edited by Arlet A, Ficat RP, Hungerford DS. Baltimore; Williams and Wilkins. 1984: 334-337.

[32] Ficat P, Arlet J, Hungerford DS (eds): *Ischaemia and Necrosis of Bone.* Baltimore, MD, Williams & Wilkins, 1980.

[33] Ficat RP: Idiopathic bone necrosis of the femoral head: Early diagnosis and treatment. *J Bone Joint Surg* 1985; 67B:3-9.

[34] Jones JP Jr: Intravascular coagulation and osteonecrosis. *Clin Orthop* 1992; 277:41-53.

[35] Jones JP Jr Fat embolism, intravascular coagulation, and osteonecrosis *Clin Orthop* 1993 Jul;(292): 294-308

[36] Jones JP Jr: Concepts of etiology and early pathogenesis of osteonecrosis. In Schafer M (ed): Instructional Course Lectures 43. *Rosemont, IL, American Academy of Orthopaedic Surgeons, 1994, pp 499-512*

[37] Babhulkar SS :Osteonecrosis of the femoral head (in young individuals) *Indian Journal of Orthopaedics* Vol.37, No.2; April 2003:77-86

[38] Yoon S,Goo Y, Kim PT, Ihn JC, Cho BC, Koo KH. Vascularized compared with nonvascularized fibular grafts for large osteonecroic lesion of the femoral head. *J Bone Joint Surg Am* 2005; 87:2012-8

[39] Dutton RO, Amstuz HC, Thomas BJ, Hedley AK Tharies surface replacement for osteonecrosis of femoral head *J Bone Joint Surgery Am* 1982; 64: 1225-1237

[40] Leung PC, Chow YY.:Reconstruction of proximal femoral defects with a vascular-pedicled graft *J Bone Joint Surg Br*, Jan 1984; 66-B: 32 – 37

[41] Leung PC: Vascular bone grafts from iliac crest *Microsurgical technique in Orthopaedics* Pho Robert WH, Butterworths; 135-144

[42] Plakseychuk AY, Bogov AA, Plakseychuk YA: vascularised Iliac crest Graft in the treatment of aseptic necrosis of femoral head; Reconstructive Microsurgery *Current Trends* Proceedings 12th Symposium International Society of Reconstructive Microsurgery, Singapore 1996: 85-87

[43] Plakseychuk AY, Kim SY, Park BC, Varitimidis SE, Rubash HE, Sotereanos DG: Vascularised compared with nonvascularised fibular bone grafting for the treatment of osteonecrosis of the femoral head. *J Bone Joint Surgery (Am)* 2003; 85:589-96.

[44] Iwata H, Torii S, Hasegawa Y, Itoh H et a.: Indications and results of vascularised pedical iliac bone graft in avascular necrosis of femoral head. *Clin Orthop*, 295:281, 1993

7

Congenital Pseudarthrosis of the Tibia: Combined Pharmacologic and Surgical Treatment Using Biphosphonate Intravenous Infusion and Bone Morphogenic Protein with Periosteal and Cancellous Autogenous Bone Grafting, Tibio-Fibular Cross Union, Intramedullary Rodding and External Fixation

Dror Paley
Paley Institute,
St. Mary's Hospital, West Palm Beach, Florida,
USA

1. Introduction

Congenital pseudarthrosis of the tibia (CPT) is one of the most challenging problems confronting pediatric orthopedic surgery. Fifty percent of cases are associated with neurofibromatosis, ten percent with fibrous dysplasia or Campanacci's osteofibrous dysplasia and forty percent are idiopathic. CPT has a tendency to refracture until skeletal maturity. Fractures can even occur in adults. The refracture incidence is reversely proportional to age. Consequently success rate of treatment methods is also age dependent and directly proportional to age. This may be related to the activity of the pathologic tissue being greater at a younger age when growth rate and metabolism are at their greatest. It may also be a function of the diameter of the bone which is smaller at a younger age and therefore more prone to fracture.

Various techniques for the management of CPT have been described. McFarland [32] described a bypass fibular graft, Boyd [3] and Boyd and Sage [4] described a double onlay graft taken from the opposite tibia combined with autologous iliac crest graft, Charnley [6] described intramedullary (IM) rods, and Sofield [41] added fragmentation and reversal of fragments. Campanacci and Zanoli [5] described a "fibula pro tibia" technique with fibular fixation to the pseudarthrosis site. Other methods include direct current or pulsed electromagnetic field, ipsilateral transfer of the fibula or contralateral free vascularized fibular transfer, circular external fixation, IM rodding, and combined external fixation and IM rodding. More recently, bone morphogenic protein (BMP) [28] and bisphosphonate therapy [20, 39] have been used. The results of all these methods have been variable. Refracture rates are high with all of these methods.

1.1 Pathology of CPT

The pathology of CPT is still unknown. During the past 100 years, a number of theories have been suggested to explain the development of the disease. Today, interest concentrates mainly on the pathologic changes of the periosteum [19]. Codivilla [8] was the first to implicate the periosteum in the pathology of CPT.

McElvenny [31] reported a markedly thickened, closely attached periosteum that caused constriction of the bone with subsequent atrophy and pseudarthrosis. The findings presented by McElvenny were echoed by Boyd [3] and Boyd and Sage [4], who suggested that CPT was caused by aggressive osteolytic fibromatosis and that those findings had been confirmed by specimens of amputated legs. Blauth et al. [1] reported the findings of a pathologic study of 10 patients with CPT and postulated that the thickened periosteum might be caused by myofibroblast overgrowth [21]. A more recent report [19] suggested that the thickened periosteum was caused by neural like cells that form a tight sheath around the small periosteal vessels causing narrowing or obliteration of vessels This results in disturbance of the blood circulation of the periosteum, which in turn results in impaired oxygen and nutrient supply of the subperiosteal bone with subsequent fracture and recalcitrant nonunion.

Cho et al. [7] studied osteoclastic and osteoblastic activities of the periosteum of seven patients with CPT compared with those of two controls. They concluded that periosteal cells stay in undifferentiated form rather than growing into abnormal cells with variable responses to BMP-2. The osteoclastic activity of the periosteum was significantly higher than that of the control, and the authors postulated that not only pathogensis of CPT but also refracture after initial healing and resorption of bone grafting are related to osteoclastic activity of the periosteum. They concluded that while the fibrous hamartoma maintains some of the mesenchymal cell phenotypes they do not undergo differentiation in response to BMP. They also showed that these cells were also more osteoclastogenic than normal tibial periosteal cells.

Schindeler et al, showed that NF1(+/-) mouse cells exhibited less osteogenic potential than NF1(+/+) cells (controls). In response to BMP the former revealed significantly less bone formation than the latter although BMP did stimulate bone formation in a heterotopic bone formation model. Co-treatment with zolidronic acid (ZA) lead to synergistic increase in bone formation in both groups. They concluded that biphosphonate-BMP combination therapy was superior to BMP therapy alone.

1.2 Periosteal grafting

Resection of hamartomatous fibrous tissue is part of many treatment protocols, but it does not ensure healing or prevent refracture. Codivilla recommended osteo-periosteal grafting more than 100 years ago [8]. Cambras (circa 1977, personal communication 1996) treated CPT with bone and periosteal grafting from the child's mother, emphasizing the role of the periosteum to cure the disease. Paley [13] proposed periosteal grafting as a treatment option in 1995 based on observations he made during his first 8 years of treating this condition [37]. Paley's periosteal grafting method was first published in a doctoral thesis by El Rossasy [14] in Egypt in 2001 and then in a book edited by Rozbruch in 2007 [13]. Paley's periosteal grafting method was used and reported on by Michael Weber [44] from Germany and Franz Grill from Austria [IPOS meeting 2006, Orlando, Florida]. A two center study combining the experience with periosteal grafting from Paley and Kocaoglu was published in 2008 by Thabet et al [42].

The Paley method of periosteal grafting described by Thabet et al was the culmination of twenty years of experience in the treatment of CPT. Paley's first report was in 1992. Followup of those and additional early Paley treated patients reported in El Rossasy's doctorate thesis demonstrated a high refracture and retreatment rate. The initial treatment was using the Ilizarov method with bone grafting of the CPT site combined with hamartoma resection. The healing rate was nearly 100% but the refracture rate was over 50%. When an IM rod was added to the Ilizarov-bone grafting treatment the refracture rate drastically dropped. Clearly the Ilizarov fixation method was excellent at obtaining union but failed to maintain union. The IM rod was excellent at maintaining union and decreasing refracture. This was also the conclusion of the multicenter EPOS study by Grill et al [17]. The efficacy of the IM rod was also increased by rodding both bones in the leg rather than just one.

Based both on the literature and on his own experience the other two factors that significantly helped decrease refracture were increasing the cross sectional area of union and eliminating angulation especially at the CPT site. Combining all of these principles Paley proposed the treatment method that was studied in the two center study reported in Thabet et al [42].

2. Paley combined pharmacologic and surgical method of treatment of CPT

Based on the new information from the recent patho-etiologic studies, Paley combined his periosteal grafting methodology [Thabet et al] with pharmacologic treatment using BMP and bisphosphonate infusion. This combination has reduced the refracture rate and accelerated the union rate as never previously observed or reported. While the union rate published in Thabet et al [42] was 100% there was a 40% refracture rate. All of these united when retreated with BMP and ZA infusion. Since the study in the 2008 publication Paley treated 15 additional cases of CPT. All united in 3-4 months and none have refractured with an average followup on average of 2 years (range 1-4 years). In addition to the previous method three changes were made to the original treatment methodology: 1) a cross union was created between the tibia and the fibula; 2) BMP was applied between the cancellous bone graft and the soft tissues as a surrounding layer including between the tibia and fibula; 3) Zolidronic acid infusion was given with the index procedure and at the time of removal of the external fixation.

2.1 Paley pharmacologic and surgical technique protocol (Fig 1)

Pharmacologic: Biphosphonate Infusion: One week prior or one week after the surgery the patient is given a Zolidronic Acid infusion intravenously (0.2mg/kg) over 30 minutes. One hour later calcium gluconate 60 mg/kg is given intravenously over the course of one hour. The patient is given 2gm elemental calcium for 7 days and Vitamin D supplementation of 400 IU for 14 days. Bone morphogenic protein which according to the FDA is considered an implant is nevertheless a protein and a growth factor. I therefore refer to its use herein as pharmacologic. Since it is applied in surgery it will be referred to there.

Surgery: The patient is placed supine, with a bump under the ipsilateral buttock, on a radiolucent table. The entire lower extremity and hemipelvis are prepped and draped free. The leg is exsanguinated and tourniquet applied. The pseudarthrosis site is approached through an anterior longitudinal incision. The thick periosteum is incised longitudinally. The periosteal incision ends at the point at which the periosteum thins to a normal thickness. Dissection between the periosteum and the surrounding soft tissues is carried out circumferentially around the tibia. Avoid injury to the anterior tibial artery laterally and the posterior tibial neurovascular bundle posterormedially.

After the hamartomatous periosteum is excised circumferentially, the proximal segment of the tibia is split by using a fine saw (Fig. 1). The split is created in such a way that it does not fracture either arm of the split. The tibia resembles the old-fashioned one-piece wooden clothes pins. The fibular pseudarthrosis is approached by dissecting posterolateral to the tibia. The fibular periosteal hamartoma is also resected.

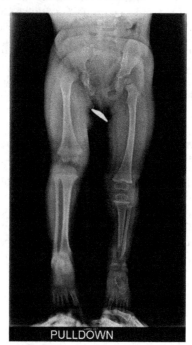

Fig. 1a. Long AP radiograph of 16 month old girl with NF and CPT left tibia with a LLD.

The distal tibial medullary canal is drilled open. The end of the distal tibia is inserted into the split of the proximal segment (occasionally when the CPT is in the mid-diaphysis instead of distal third the distal fragment is split the proximal is invanginated into the distal split). The proximal fibula is invaginated into a similar split of the distal fibula. The tibia and fibula are shortened by 1 to 2 cm. In a previously unoperated case, the only bone resection that is performed is the minimal required to open the medullary canal. In a previously operated case there may be dead bone present which should be resected. To determine what bone is alive vs dead, the tourniquet is released and all non bleeding bone is resected. A high speed burr is helpful in causing the bone to bleed while doing controlled debridement.

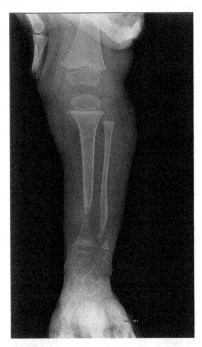

Fig. 1b. AP of the tibia before surgery.

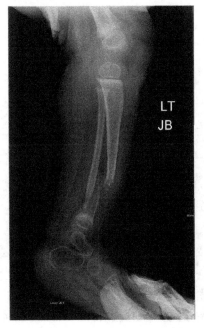

Fig. 1c. Lateral of the tibia before surgery.

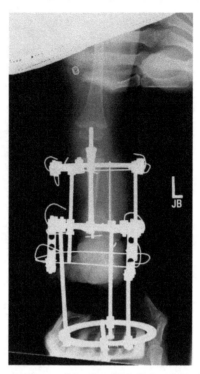

Fig. 1d. AP of the tibia after surgery with telescopic IM rod in place and Ilizarov device in place. Note the walking extension on the external fixator that allows for equalization of the leg length and weightbearing during treatment.

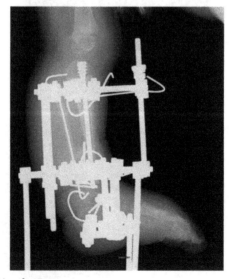

Fig. 1e. Lateral of the tibia after surgery.

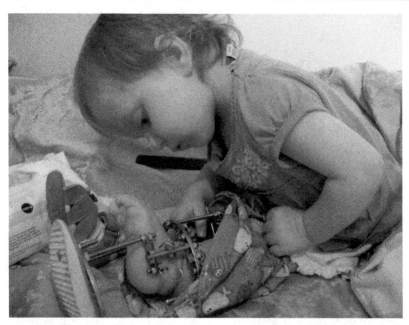

Fig. 1f. Photograph of the child with the external fixator on. She had little pain and few pin
site problems.

An IM rod is inserted across the CPT site. The implant used depends on the age and
diameter of the CPT bone. One can use a Kirschner wire or Steinmann pin in very-small-
diameter bone or a Rush rod or flexible titanium rod in larger diameter bones. The rod can
be inserted from distal to proximal via the medial malleolus or from proximal to distal
crossing the proximal physis. The distal to proximal technique is much more difficult
because the medial malleolus is very medially located relative to the mid-diaphyseal line.
There is a tendency to create a lateral translation deformity if the rod is not properly
molded. Most recently, we have used the Paley-modified Fassier-Duval telescopic IM nail
system (Pega Medical, Inc. Laval, Quebec, Canada) from proximal to distal. The Paley
modification of this nail allows locking into the distal tibial epiphysis using a threaded
1.6mm Kirschner wire. It is preferable to avoid rodding across the ankle joint to prevent
stiffness of the ankle joint and permanent poor push-off strength [23]. The fibula should be
rodded retrograde from the lateral malleolus using a wire of between 1-2mm in diameter. It
is important to coordinate the rodding and shortening of the tibia and fibula so that one
bone does not impede the shortening of the other bone.

An incision is then made along the iliac crest. The apophysis is split and the medial
periosteum with the iliacus muscle reflected medially off the ilium. The cancellous bone
between the cortical tables of the ilium is harvested. In young children this will not yield
enough bone. Therefore the tables can be split with a sharp osteotome towards the roof of
the acetabulum. There is a large amount of cancellous bone located in the supra-acetabular
region. This can be reached with a curette after splitting the tables using image intensifier
guidance. Even in a one year old child there is ample cancellous bone to be found in the
supra-acetabular region. The bone in the donor site reconstitutes after the harvest.

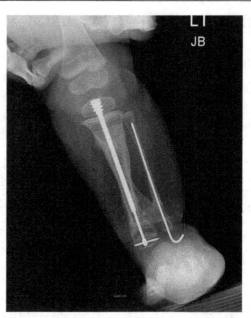

Fig. 1g. Long AP radiograph standing showing the remaining LLD that will be treated at a later date. The tibia and fibular are healed.

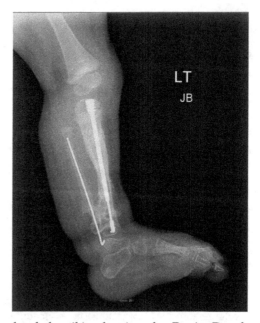

Fig. 1h. AP radiograph of the tibia showing the Fassier-Duval with the distal Paley modificaiton (locking to the distal epiphysis with a threaded k-wire). The tibia and fibula show a cross union and both bones show are now solidly united.

The best place to procure periosteum is beneath the iliacus muscle. If more is needed then the periosteum beneath the gluteal muscles can also be harvested by reflecting the lateral half of the apophysis off of the lateral table of the ilium. A knife is used to incise the periosteum in as long and as wide a rectangular piece as possible. The periosteum is then separated from the overlying muscle. The periosteum immediately shrinks to a quarter its original size. To restore some of its size, it is placed through the skin graft mesher and expanded. The meshed periosteum is expanded and then wrapped around the invaginated bone ends of the pseudarthrosis site. It is important that the cambium layer face the bone. To apply the periosteum two sutures can be tied to two of the corners of the rectangular graft. The graft is then pulled around the posterior aspect of the bone and sutured to itself. The same is done to the fibular pseudarthrosis site. The cancellous bone graft is then placed circumferentially around the pseudarthrosis site and filled into the space between the two bones. Finally bone morphogenic protein (BMP-2; Infuse, Medtronics, Memphis, TN) is placed around the bone graft between the bone graft and the surrounding soft tissues. The bone grafting and BMP are especially located in the space between the tibia and fibula to create a cross union. The wound is then closed over a Hemovac drain.

After closure, an Ilizarov all-wire frame is applied to the limb. This requires three wires in the proximal metaphysis (two counter opposed olive wires and one smooth wire), three distal wires, and foot fixation. The wires should not be in contact with the IM rod. A walking ring is applied postoperatively so that the patient does not have to bear weight on the foot. The main purpose of the fixator is to give rotatory control and stability to the pseudarthrosis site.

3. Post-operative management

The patient's wound is checked two weeks after surgery. Radiographs are obtained at 6 and 12 weeks after surgery. The bone is usually united by 12 weeks after surgery. The external fixator can be removed once radiographic union is confirmed and a long leg walking cast applied. After removal and after the swelling decreases the patient should be measured for a knee-ankle-foot orthotic with a free knee hinge and a solid ankle. As the patient grows the brace should be remade. Eventually (over age 6), an articulated ankle is added. As the patient gets older the length of the brace is reduced. Then the thigh cuff is removed and only a total contact articulated AFO or PTB brace used. When the patient is older (over age 10 a gator brace (no foot part with lateral and medial malleolar flanges) is used. Brace wear at all times including during sleep and swimming is used until skeletal maturity. The only time the brace is taken off is for bathing and for physical therapy. Sports and other activities are allowed while wearing the brace. Patients treated engaged in wrestling, surfing, skiing, cycling, etc.

The IM rod should be changed as needed. If a telescopic rod is used it should be changed to a larger diameter rod as the patient grows. Since the length of the bone doubles from age 3 in girls and 4 years old in boys till skeletal maturity, the telescopic rod has to be changed once before maturity and once before age 4. Zolidronic acid infusion should be given with each rodding surgery.

Hemiepiphysiodesis is also performed if a valgus ankle or knee is present. The presence of the rod does not impede the use of a hemi-epiphysiodesis screw plate device.

4. Discussion

The natural history of CPT is recalcitrant nonunion, atrophy of the bone and the leg, progressive LLD and deformity, and recurrent refracture even after union is acheived in surgery [3, 4, 22, 29, 33]. The primary objective of treatment for CPT is to obtain union. The secondary objective is to maintain union. In addition, many associated deformities of length and angulation should be addressed in the comprehensive management of CPT. Therefore, unless all patients have reached skeletal maturity, the refracture rate reported is always lower than actual [3, 4, 33].

The main surgical options for treatment of CPT are vascularized fibular grafting, IM stabilization, external fixation with a circular frame, and amputation [9–11, 17, 18, 26, 30, 35]. Electric stimulation has also been studied [37, 38]

Paley et al. [35] presented a report of 15 patients who had 16 tibiae with congenital pseudarthrosis. The mean patient age was 8 years, the rate of union was 94% in 15 patients with Ilizarov frames, refracture occurred in five tibiae (31%), and the mean followup duration was 4 years.

Boero et al. [2] presented a report of 21 patients with neurofibromatosis treated with Ilizarov frames. The mean patient age was 8.8 years. The primary union rate was achieved in 17 of 21 (81%) patients. Refracture occurred in four of the 17 patients (19%), and the minimum followup duration was 2 years.

The European Paediatric Orthopaedic Society (EPOS) multicenter study [17] of 340 patients with CPT reported a 75% healing rate achieved with Ilizarov external fixation and recommended the use of prophylactic IM rodding to prevent refracture.

In a series of 17 tibiae with CPT treated by Paley and Herzenberg, half of which were followed up to skeletal maturity, the mean patient age was 8 years, union was obtained in 100% of the patients, and refracture occurred in 68% when the Ilizarov device without IM rodding was used [14]. When IM rodding was combined with external fixation, the refracture rate dropped to 29%.

Ohnishi et al. [34] reported 73 cases that were treated with different treatment protocols: 26 with Ilizarov fixation, 25 with vascularized fibular grafting, seven with the combination of the previous two techniques, six with IM rodding combined with free bone grafting, five with plating and grafting, and the remaining four with different treatment protocols. The average patient age was 5 years. Union was achieved in all patients treated with Ilizarov fixation (four experienced refracture), 22 of 25 (88%) patients treated with free vascularized fibular grafting (one experienced refracture), and all patients treated with both fibular grafting and Ilizarov fixation.

IM rodding is an alternative treatment option to achieve and maintain union, although the reported results are variable. Joseph and Mathew [24] reported 14 skeletally immature patients treated with IM rodding and double onlay autogenous bone grafting from the opposite tibia. The mean patient age was 4.5 years, the union rate was 86%, the mean followup duration was 3 years, and the refracture rate was 21% (three of 14).

Johnston [23] presented a report of 23 patients treated with different techniques of IM rodding and grafting. The mean patient age was 2 years 4 months, the mean followup duration was 9 years, the primary union rate was 87%, and 13% had persistent nonunion and bad outcomes. The author noted that two important factors for the best outcome for patients with CPT were perfect limb alignment and the use of IM rods to achieve union, prevent refracture, and maintain alignment.

Kim and Weinstein [27] presented a report of 11 patients with 12 tibiae with congenital pseudarthrosis treated with IM rodding and free bone grafting. The mean patient age at the time of the index operation was 2.5 years. Four of the 11 patients healed after the primary index operation. Two of the four experienced refracture; one healed with a long lower limb cast, and the other healed after the index operation was repeated. The other seven did not heal after the index operation. Four of them achieved healing after undergoing multiple surgical procedures (one required free vascularized fibular grafting, and three required repeated IM rodding and grafting; one of the three had nonunion, one needed Syme amputation, and one had a failed Sofield procedure). Healing could not be achieved in the other three patients (two underwent below-knee amputation, and one had persistent nonunion at the latest followup visit). Kim concluded that IM rodding provides more predictable results in cases of late-onset pseudarthrosis.

Dobbs et al. [9, 10] reported the long-term followup (mean followup duration, 14.2 years) of 21 patients with CPT (mean patient age, 5.1 years) treated with IM rodding and bone grafting. The primary union rate was 86% (18 patients), and three patients required additional bone grafting to achieve union. Twelve patients (57%) experienced refracture, and five (24%) required amputation.

Free vascularized fibular grafting had been described by several authors as a good option for acheiving union in patients with CPT, although it is associated with many drawbacks, including nonunion, refracture, and recurrent nonunion at one site of the graft end [11, 16, 25, 45]. Angular deformity of the affected tibia (valgus or anterior bowing) has been reported. The deformities usually are progressive and require further treatment [15, 25, 45]. Donor site morbidity, such as progressive ankle valgus with proximal migration of the distal fibula, is another problem associated with vascularized fibular grafting [15, 25, 45]. The tibiofibular synostosis can only delay but not prevent ankle valgus [15].

Weiland et al. [45] presented a report of 19 patients with a 95% union rate. Initial failure to achieve union occurred in 26% (five of 19 patients), and those patients required secondary procedures to achieve union (four healed and one underwent amputation).

Gilbert [16] reported the long-term followup of 29 patients who had CPT treated with microvascular fibular grafting, all of whom had reached skeletal maturity. The union rate was 94% with a mean healing time of 6 months. The mean patient age at the time of the index operaion was 5.5 years, the refracture rate was 14%, and the reccurence rate was 7%. Donor site morbidity occurred in 24%, tibial deformity (valgus and anterior bowing) occurred in 24%, progressive LLD occurred in 7%, and no ampuation was recorded.

The EPOS study [26, 39] reported a healing rate of 61% (19 of 31 patients). Seven of the 19 healed patients required additional procedures, such as grafting, plating, or IM rodding. The remaining 12 healed after the primary treatment and did not require additional surgery. Three patients (10%) required amputations, seven (23%) had not healed, and five (16%) experienced fracture of the transfered fibula.

Toh et al. [43] reported seven cases of CPT treated with vascularized fibular graft, with a mean followup duration of 12.1 years. Casting or monolateral external fixation was used in the first cases; an Ilizarov fixator was used as a postopertative immobilization tool in one case. The author concluded that the best outcome can be acheived with combined vascularized fibular grafting and Ilizarov external fixation as a method of postopertaive fixation.

El-Gamal et al. [12] reported three cases of CPT treated with vascularized fibular grafting combined with Ilizarov fixation to distract the fibular graft to correct LLD with a single operation. They called it 'telescoping vascularized fibular graft'. The mean patient age was 9 years, and the mean followup duration was 2 years. Union was achieved in all cases. One patient experienced refracture, and another patient experienced ankle valgus of the affected site.

Amputation is an option in cases of CPT [18, 30]. Its incidence varies from series to series. McCarthy [30] noted that foot condition, number of operations, and severity of LLD are the factors that determine the need for amputation.

Pharmacologic therapuetic solutions for CPT recently have become available: BMP-2, BMP-7 and bisphosphonate therapy (ZA) [20, 28, 40]. Lee et al. [28] reported five cases of CPT treated with BMP-7 combined with corticocancellous allograft and IM rodding combined with external fixation. The mean patient age was 6 years, and the mean followup duration was 14 months. The authors conluded that the use of recombinant human BMP-7 is not enough to overcome the poor healing environment associated with CPT. Little and colleagues [20, 40] used bisphosphonate (ZA) for patients with CPT to control the activity of osteoclasts to promote union and prevent the bone graft from resorption.

Thabet, Paley, Kocoaglu et al [42] conducted a retrospective study of 20 patients with CPT who were treated with periosteal grafting and bone grafting combined with IM rodding of the tibia and fibula and circular external fixation by the senior authors between 1997 and 2006 at two centers. The mean age at the index operation was 4.2 years (age range, 1–11.3 years). Eleven patients (55%) had neurofibromatosis, in seven patients (35%) the condition was idiopathic, and two patients (10%) had osteofibrous dysplasia. Twelve patients (60%) had no previous surgery, and eight patients (40%) had undergone at least one unsuccessful operation (range, 0–14). All patients had established pseudarthrosis. Union was achieved in all patients (100%). The mean time spent in external fixation was 5.2 months (range, 3–12 months). Limb lengthening was achieved in 12 patients. The mean lengthening amount was 2.5 cm (range, 0–7 cm); epiphysiodesis of the opposite side was performed in one patient.

Refracture occurred in eight patients: six experienced one refracture each, and two experienced two refractures each. Six of the eight patients with refracture had fibular pseudarthrosis. The mean time between the index operation and refracture was 2.3 years (range, 1–5.8 years), and the mean time between the index operation and second refracture was 4.7 years. The mean age at the index operation of patients who experienced refracture was 4 years (range, 1–7.3 years). The mean followup duration was 4.3 years (range, 2–10.7 years). All of the refractures were treated and all healed with surgery.

Most recently Paley studied 15 cases treated by the combined pharmacologic and surgical management method described above. The age range was from 1-10 years (mean 4 years). All patients united. There were no refractures. The average followup was 2 years (range 1-4).

Based on these results there is reason to believe that combining BMP and bisphosphonate treatment in clinical practice is a useful adjunct as was shown in the animal model [40]. In a review of CPT, Johnston and Birch [22] advocated using BMP as an adjuvant treatment in all primary and recalcitrant cases. Despite optimism with the use of BMP, one must also consider theoretical risk of tumorgenesis because BMP stimulates the RAS pathway, which is also a tumor pathway. Patients with CPT have a propensity for both benign and malignant tumors. Although there has never been a report of such a complication, it should be discussed with patients since rhBMP is not FDA-approved for children or for CPT.

The Paley method of combined pharmacologic and surgical management is a shotgun approach to management of this potentially devastating problem. It optimizes the mechanical [33]and biologic environment for the CPT. It is impossible to identify which factor is more important for the healing of CPT since no control group or comparison study has been done. Since this is a rare disease and failure is devastating it is more important to have a successful method than to be certain which component of the treatment regimen is the most important to achieving successful union. As newer pharmacologic therapeutics and better understanding of the patho-etiology of this disease occur, the combined pharmacologic surgical technique will morph to include newer technologies and therapeutics. Meanwhile the combination treatment; hamartoma resection, periosteal grafting, bone grafting, internal rodding, external fixation, tibio-fibular cross union, BMP and bisphosphonate pharmacologic manipulation are the best current combination treatment for CPT.

5. References

[1] Blauth M, Harms D, Schmidt D, Blauth W. Light- and electron-microscopic studies in congenital pseudarthrosis. *Arch Orthop Trauma Surg.* 1984;103:269–277.

[2] Boero S, Catagni M, Donzelli O, Facchini R, Frediani PV. Congenital pseudarthrosis of the tibia associated with neurofibromatosis-1: treatment with Ilizarov's device. *J Pediatr Orthop.* 1997;17:675–684.

[3] Boyd HB. Pathology and natural history of congenital pseudarthrosis of the tibia. *Clin Orthop Relat Res.* 1982;166:5–13.

[4] Boyd HB, Sage FP. Congenital pseudarthrosis of the tibia. *J Bone Joint Surg Am.* 1958;40:1245–1270.

[5] Campanacci M, Zanoli S. Double tibiofibular synostosis (fibula pro tibia) for non-union and delayed union of the tibia: end-result review of one hundred seventy-one cases. *J Bone Joint Surg Am.* 1966;48:44–56.

[6] Charnley J. Congenital pseudarthrosis of the tibia treated by intramedullary nail. *J Bone Joint Surg Am.* 1956;38:283–290.

[7] Cho T-J, Seo JB, Lee HR, Chung CY, Choi IH. Biologic characteristics of fibrous hamartoma from congenital pseudarthrosis of the tibia associated with neurofibroumatosis type 1. J Bone Joint Surg Am 2008; 90 (12): 2735-44.

[8] Codivilla A. On the cure of the congenital pseudoarthrosis of the tibia by means of periosteal transplanation. *J Bone Joint Surg Am.* 1906;s2-4:163–169.

[9] Dobbs MB, Rich MM, Gordon JE, Szymanski DA, Schoenecker PL. Use of an intramedullary rod for treatment of congenital pseudarthrosis of the tibia: a long-term followup study. *J Bone Joint Surg Am.* 2004;86:1186–1197.

[10] Dobbs MB, Rich MM, Gordon JE, Szymanski DA, Schoenecker PL. Use of an intramedullary rod for the treatment of congenital pseudarthrosis of the tibia: surgical technique. *J Bone Joint Surg Am.* 2005;87(Suppl 1):33–40.

[11] Dormans JP, Krajbich JI, Zuker R, Demuynk M. Congenital pseudarthrosis of the tibia: treatment with free vascularized fibular grafts. *J Pediatr Orthop.* 1990;10:623–628.

[12] El-Gammal TA, El-Sayed A, Kotb MM. Telescoping vascularized fibular graft: a new method for treatment of congenital tibial pseudarthrosis with severe shortening. *J Pediatr Orthop B.* 2004;13:48–56.

[13] El-Rosasy MA, Paley D, Herzenberg JE. Congenital pseudarthrosis of the tibia. In: Rozbruch SR, Ilizarov S, eds. *Limb Lengthening and Reconstruction Surgery.* New York: Informa Healthcare; 2007:485–493.

[14] El-Rosasy MA, Paley D, Herzenberg JE. Ilizarov techniques for the management of congenital pseudarthrosis of the tibia (PhD Thesis). Tanta, Egypt: Tanta University Press; 2001.

[15] Fragnière B, Wicart P, Mascard E, Dubousset J. Prevention of ankle valgus after vascularized fibular grafts in children. *Clin Orthop Relat Res.* 2003;408:245–251.

[16] Gilbert A, Brockman R. Congenital pseudarthrosis of the tibia: long-term followup of 29 cases treated by microvascular bone transfer. *Clin Orthop Relat Res.* 1995;314:37–44.

[17] Grill F, Bollini G, Dungl P, Fixsen J, Hefti F, Ippolito E, Romanus B, Tudisco C, Wientroub S. Treatment approaches for congenital pseudarthrosis of tibia: results of the EPOS multicenter study: European Paediatric Orthopaedic Society (EPOS). *J Pediatr Orthop B.* 2000;9:75–89.

[18] Guille JT, Kumar SJ, Shah A. Spontaneous union of a congenital pseudarthrosis of the tibia after Syme amputation. *Clin Orthop Relat Res.* 1998;351:180–185.

[19] Hermanns-Sachweh B, Senderek J, Alfer J, Klosterhalfen B, Büttner R, Füzesi L, Weber M. Vascular changes in the periosteum of congenital pseudarthrosis of the tibia. *Pathol Res Pract.* 2005;201:305–312.

[20] Högler W, Yap F, Little D, Ambler G, McQuade M, Cowell CT. Short-term safety assessment in the use of intravenous zoledronic acid in children. *J Pediatr.* 2004;145:701–704.

[21] Ippolito E, Corsi A, Grill F, Wientroub S, Bianco P. Pathology of bone lesions associated with congenital pseudarthrosis of the leg. *J Pediatr Orthop B.* 2000;9:3–10.

[22] Jacobsen ST, Crawford AH, Millar EA, Steel HH. The Syme amputation in patients with congenital pseudarthrosis of the tibia. *J Bone Joint Surg Am.* 1983;65:533–537.

[23] Johnston CE II. Congenital pseudarthrosis of the tibia: results of technical variations in the Charnley-Williams procedure. *J Bone Joint Surg Am.* 2002;84:1799–1810.

[24] Joseph B, Mathew G. Management of congenital pseudarthrosis of the tibia by excision of the pseudarthrosis, onlay grafting, and intramedullary nailing. *J Pediatr Orthop B.* 2000;9:16–23.

[25] Kanaya F, Tsai TM, Harkess J. Vascularized bone grafts for congenital pseudarthrosis of the tibia. *Microsurgery.* 1996;17:459–469.

[26] Keret D, Bollini G, Dungl P, Fixsen J, Grill F, Hefti F, Ippolito E, Romanus B, Tudisco C, Wientroub S. The fibula in congenital pseudoarthrosis of the tibia: the EPOS multicenter study: European Paediatric Orthopaedic Society (EPOS). *J Pediatr Orthop B.* 2000;9:69–74.

[27] Kim HW, Weinstein SL. Intramedullary fixation and bone grafting for congenital pseudarthrosis of the tibia. *Clin Orthop Relat Res.* 2002;405:250–257.

[28] Lee FY, Sinicropi SM, Lee FS, Vitale MG, Roye DP Jr, Choi IH. Treatment of congenital pseudarthrosis of the tibia with recombinant human bone morphogenetic protein-7 (rhBMP-7): a report of five cases. *J Bone Joint Surg Am.* 2006;88:627–633.

[29] Masserman RL, Peterson HA, Bianco AJ Jr. Congenital pseudarthrosis of the tibia: a review of the literature and 52 cases from the Mayo Clinic. *Clin Orthop Relat Res.* 1974;99:140–145.

[30] McCarthy RE. Amputation for congenital pseudarthrosis of the tibia: indications and techniques. *Clin Orthop Relat Res.* 1982;166:58–61.

[31] McElvenny RT. Congenital pseudarthrosis of the tibia: the findings in one case and a suggestion as to possible etiology and treatment. *Q Bull Northwest Univ Med Sch.* 1949;23:413–423.

[32] McFarland B. Pseudarthrosis of the tibia in childhood. *J Bone Joint Surg Br.* 1951;33:36–46.

[33] Morrissy RT. Congenital pseudarthrosis of the tibia: factors that affect results. *Clin Orthop Relat Res.* 1982;166:21–27.

[34] Ohnishi I, Sato W, Matsuyama J, Yajima H, Haga N, Kamegaya M, Minami A, Sato M, Yoshino S, Oki T, Nakamura K. Treatment of congenital pseudarthrosis of the tibia: a multicenter study in Japan. *J Pediatr Orthop.* 2005;25:219–224.

[35] Paley D, Catagni M, Argnani F, Prevot J, Bell D, Armstrong P. Treatment of congenital pseudoarthrosis of the tibia using the Ilizarov technique. *Clin Orthop Relat Res.* 1992;280:81–93.

[36] Paley D, Congenital Pseudarthrosis: Management. *PanArabOrthopaediCongress Muscat, Oman* Sept 11-14, 1995

[37] Paterson DC, Lewis GN, Cass CA. Treatment of congenital pseudarthrosis of the tibia with direct current stimulation. *Clin Orthop Relat Res.* 1980;148:129–135.

[38] Paterson DC, Simonis RB. Electrical stimulation in the treatment of congenital pseudarthrosis of the tibia. *J Bone Joint Surg Br.* 1985;67:454–462.

[39] Romanus B, Bollini G, Dungl P, Fixsen J, Grill F, Hefti F, Ippolito E, Tudisco C, Wientroub S. Free vascular fibular transfer in congenital pseudoarthrosis of the tibia: results of the EPOS multicenter study: European Paediatric Orthopaedic Society (EPOS). *J Pediatr Orthop B.* 2000;9:90–93.

[40] Schindeler A, Ramachandran M, Godfrey C, Morse A, McDonald M, Mikulec K, Little DG. Modeling bone morphogenetic protein and bisphosphonate combination therapy in wild-type and Nf1 haploinsufficient mice. *J Orthop Res.* 2008;26:65–74.

[41] Sofield HA. Congenital pseudarthrosis of the tibia. *Clin Orthop Relat Res.* 1971;76:33–42.

[42] Thabet AM, Paley D, Kocaoglu M, Eralp L, Herzenberg JE, Ergin ON. Periosteal grafting for congenital pseudarthrosis of the tibia: a preliminary report. *Clin Orthop Relat Res.* 2008;466:2981-94. *Epub* 2008 Oct 25.

[43] Toh S, Harata S, Tsubo K, Inoue S, Narita S. Combining free vascularized fibula graft and the Ilizarov external fixator: recent approaches to congenital pseudarthrosis of the tibia. *J Reconstr Microsurg.* 2001;17:497–508.

[44] Weber M., Congenital pseudarthrosis of the tibia redefined: congenital crural segemental dysplasia. In: Rozbruch SR, Ilizarov S, eds. *Limb Lengthening and Reconstruction Surgery.* New York: Informa Healthcare; 2007:495–509.

[45] Weiland AJ, Weiss AP, Moore JR, Tolo VT. Vascularized fibular grafts in the treatment of congenital pseudarthrosis of the tibia. *J Bone Joint Surg Am.* 1990;72:654–662.

8

Treatment of Distal Radius Bone Defects with Injectable Calcium Sulphate Cement

Deng Lei, Ma Zhanzhong, Yang Huaikuo, Xue Lei and Yang Gongbo

Orthopaedic Department,
Beijing XiYuan Hospital,
China Academy of Chinese Medical Science,
China

1. Introduction

In the treatment of distal radius fractures, bone grafting for subchondral bone defects is often used in order to avoid articular surface collapse and radial shortening. At present, the bone graft materials used regularly include autogenous bone, allogeneic bone or heterogenous bone and synthetic materials. Autogenous bone graft has been the gold standard for bone grafting and is the ideal implant bone substitute, but its source is limited[1] [2].Moreover, opening reduction to expose the fracture segment and the donor site of bone will increase blood loss, surgery time and the possibility of infection. Allogeneic bone, although solving the problem of insufficient amount, has the disadvantage of the lack of sources and has the potential for immune response, infection and re-fracture [3][4]. Synthetic calcium sulphate graft has the advantage of good biocompatibility, it is biodegradable and injectable and will set in situ, which makes it an excellent choice for the clinical application of the treatment of distal radius fracture, particularly suitable to be implanted by injection. Its' relatively rapid resorption time and complete resorption will minimize the risks associated with any intra-articular migration, which could be a problem with the much slower resorbing calcium phosphate cements. The authors present a retrospective analysis of the clinical outcome on the treatment of distal radius fractures using calcium sulphate cement.

2. Material and operating technique

2.1 Patient selection

Over a period of four years, from January 2006 to January 2010, data from 60 patients was reviewed; 42 males and 18 females, ages from 46-68 years old (mean age 56 years old). Fractures were classified to A3 (12 cases), C2 (28 cases) and C3 (20 cases) using AO classification and all had some degree of subchondral bone defects. There were 8 cases treated with closing reduction and 52 cases treated with external fixation. In all cases fractures were implanted with calcium sulfate cement (Stimulan Kit, Biocomposites Ltd., UK) without autogenous bone graft.

2.2 Calcium sulphate cement filling

After appropriate fixation, the size of the bone defect was preliminarily measured before cement injection. Puncture needles were inserted into the gaps of fracture defect under fluoroscopic control. Once the needle position was satisfactory the calcium sulphate powder and diluent were mixed. The paste was extruded into the defect cavity until full when viewed under fluoroscopy. The implantation was made in different directions to access all gaps. In all cases 3 - 5cc of paste was used and the whole implantation procedure was completed within 6 minutes.

3. Clinical result

Fractures healed in all cases. All patients were followed up for 4 to 18 months (mean 8 months) and X-ray images were taken for review. The study found that callus appeared in all cases within 2 to 4 months. Most of the calcium sulphate had absorbed within 2 months and all was completely absorbed in 3 months post surgery.

X-ray images for 57 patients demonstrated that the reduction of the fracture was stable and satisfactory, with no fracture side collapse and/or displacement found. 3 cases showed slight collapse which may be a result of the adjustment of the external fixator too early after the surgery.

No foreign body reactions or infection were found in all 60 patients. No complications such as pin loosening dislocation of fixators, injury of blood vessels and radial nerves, pin track infections occurred. According to Mcbride scoring, the results were excellent in 50 cases, good in 7 cases, fair in 1 case and poor in 2 cases, the excellent and good rate being 95%. Two cases had traumatic arthritis and 1 case had wrist joint stiffness.

4. Complications

Significant complications have been rare. In most cases of this group, the external fixators were applied. One case showed slight collapse since corrected the external fixator earlier after reduction, which may be a result of the adjustment of the external fixator too early after the surgery (Fig 1,2). The authors recommend that correcting the external fixator should pay attention to avoid the distal end re-displacement and collapse.

Two patients had radial shortening. Yang D.F[5] analyzed the causes of postoperative radial shortening includes: (1) patients older than 60 years; (2) severe osteoporosis; (3) preoperative displacement and comminuted fractures; (4) inappropriate fixation methods; (5) inadequate bone graft; (6) premature load. The key points to enhance the treatment outcomes include precise judgement of the fracture type and bone quality, sufficient bone graft, firmly fixed after anatomical reduction and an appropriate plan for early loadless functional exercise. Traumatic arthritis may be avoided or delayed if the above-mentioned causes can be taken into consideration or preventive measures can be taken. (Fig 3)

Sometimes the calcium sulphate cement out of the bone defect area, even outside of the medullary cavity of bone, and the cement may be overflow into soft tissue. It may be a stimulant to irritate cellulitis of soft tissue. Kelly Cynthia[6] et al reported in a prospective, nonrandomized, multicenter study, and 109 patients with bone defects were treated with a surgical grade calcium sulfate preparation as a bone graft substitute. There were 13 complications; however, only four (3.6%) were attributable to the product. Joseph[7] et al reported complications included persistent nonunion (four patients), wound drainage (five patients), wound drainage and cellulitis (one patient) and cellulitis alone (one patient).

In operation, surgery should pay attention to avoid the cement out and into the soft tissue. If the cement mass close to the major blood vessel and nerve, getting them out by surgery recommended.

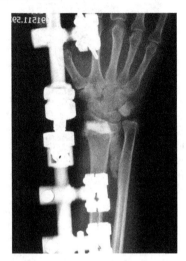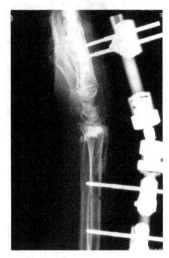

Fig. 1. Female, 68 years old. Postoperative anteroposterior and lateral image shown good alignment.

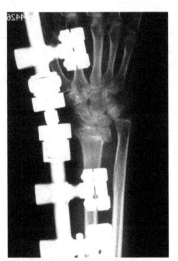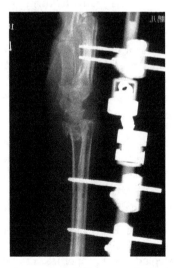

Fig. 2. At 8 weeks after operation, the picture showed collapse and shortening of distal radius which may be a result of the adjustment of the external fixator too early after the surgery.

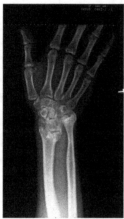 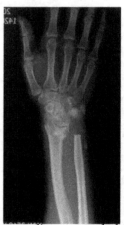

Fig. 3. Male, 54 years old. Distal radius fracture and plaster splint was used after injury. No bone grafting and fixator were giving. Three months later, distal radius collapse and malunion, and traumatic arthritis occurred. Distal ulna-ectomy was given for improve the function of the wrist.

5. Discussion

The routine clinical treatment of distal radius fractures is closed reduction and/or external fixation. As the fracture is commonly to the metaphyseal joint, particularly in the elderly, it is easy to cause fracture displacement, collapse, distal radioulnar joint instability and shortening of the radius following reduction because of unstable fixation. Although open reduction can help reduce the occurrence of fracture re-displacement with internal fixation, it is difficult to achieve anatomical reduction on complex and comminuted fractures. Also there is risk of infection. The ability to carry out closed reduction, effectively maintaining bone fragment stability and good alignment of the distal radioulnar joint is a key issue. In recent years, many surgeons prefer to use external fixation plus metaphyseal bone grafting to treat distal radius bone fractures[8,9,10], such as leverage reduction and bone graft. intramedullary implant with bone graft, insert pin with bone graft etc, and this technique has achieved satisfactory results. The authors retrospectively analyzed 60 patients who sustained such fractures and showed that external fixation combined with minimally invasive injection of calcium sulphate bone cement is an excellent method to treat distal radius bone defects.

5.1 Synthetic calcium sulfate cement

In recent years, many biomedical scientists have carried out research to find the ideal bone substitute with mechanical strength, excellent biocompatibility, and with osteoconductive and osteoinductive properties. The bone substitute should be fully biodegradable with an absorption rate similar to the rate of new bone formation. Commonly used bone graft substitutes include heterogeneous bone, polymers and biologically active ceramics (hydroxyapatite and tricalcium phosphate) which have no osteoinductive activity and some implant material combined with BMP claiming osteoinductive activity. The characteristics of calcium sulfate can meet the criteria of an ideal bone substitute and is therefore of value in clinical application.

For larger bone defects caused by trauma, the routine treatment involves bone grafting. When filling with calcium sulfate or other synthetic bone materials (pellet or granules are used commonly), the method of implantation is the same as the traditional bone grafting. However, for irregular shaped defects, pellets/granules tend to be filled by an open procedure, and also are difficult to fill into every corner. Only tightly filling can maximize the likelihood of consolidation of fracture fragments, by providing an effective scaffold for bone conduction. As calcium sulphate cement can be shaped and adapted to any irregular shapes of defect, it can overcome the disadvantages presented by granular materials. In addition, when set, it helps the defect area resists loading forces. In this study, all 60 patients with distal radial fractures combined with subchondral bone defects were treated by using injectable calcium sulphate cement to fill the defects. It was simple to inject the calcium sulphate cement and the results were satisfactory. In addition, because of the use of a minimally invasive technique, it minimized disturbing the fracture site blood supply and interference with the fracture region, and supported the biological basis of fracture healing as scheduled. Bavonratanavech[11] et al has also recently reported on the use of injectable cement (calcium phosphate) to treat fresh distal radius fractures, and concluded that it has the advantages of convenient use of injection, supporting metaphysis, reducing both operation time and the risk of infection with reliable healing results. The authors would not recommend any adjustment to the external fixation equipment between 1.5 and 2 months after surgery as the mean absorption time of the injectable calcium sulphate cement was 2.5 months and there is a potential risk of displacement of fracture segments prior to healing.

In this study, one case presented with a slight distal radius collapse at 6 weeks after surgery when adjusting the external fixator. It was speculated it may be related with the time of adjustment in addition to the serious degree of comminuted fractures and insufficient cement filling.

Lobenhoffer[12] et al retrospectively analyzed 26 cases sustaining unstable tibial plateau fractures. 25 cases were open reduction with plates and screws for fixation and one case was closed reduction. In all cases calcium phosphate cement (Norian SRS, Synthes) was injected into the condyle bone defects. Mean follow-up time for all cases was 19.7 months. In all cases no re-displaced fracture was evident. The authors believed that the synthetic bone cement used has the advantage of high safety, good supporting strength and avoiding the need for autogenous bone graft. The cement could be arbitrarily shaped and completely fill the defect. In addition treatment allowed passive exercises of the limbs at an average of 4.5 weeks after surgery.

Calcium sulphate is not commonly expected to show bone induction ability as it is considered a simple inorganic salt. However, Walsh [13] et al used immunostaining methods and found that it increased the amount of BMP (bone morphogenic protein), IgG (immunoglobulin G), PDGF (platelet derived growth factor) and TGF-β (transforming growth factor-beta) and other important factors in new bone formation sites. Following implantion of calcium sulfate in bone defects, it may promote the fracture healing process through a variety of ways and Gitelis[14] reported that calcium sulphate was a good substitute for autogenous bone. In this study, results have indicated that although the calcium sulfate was absorbed in 2 or 3 months, strong bone healing capability was observed. Whether calcium sulphate possesses an osteoinductive function explaining why excellent bone healing is achieved in these patients is yet to be determined. Further *in-vitro* and *in-vivo* studies are required.

Distal radius fractures, especially classified by AO as A3, B3 and C-type of metaphyseal cancellous bone defect and articular surface collapse, were a good indication to use injectable calcium sulphate cement. In the author's experience, this injection method is suitable for patients who have collapse of the articular surface and a defect larger than 0.5cm and with the gap of cavities less than 2.5cm. An open reduction would be needed if the defect was greater than 2.5cm. The injection needle is usually introduced from the dorsal side, and great care should be taken to avoid over injection of cement to prevent neurovascular compression in the palm side (Fig 4, 5).

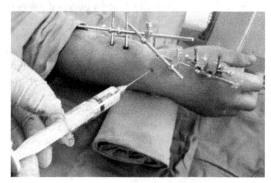

Fig. 4. The injection needle is usually introduced from the dorsal side, and great care should be taken to avoid over injection of cement to prevent neurovascular compression in the palm side.

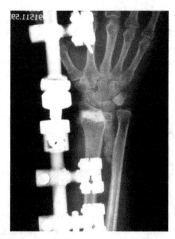

Fig. 5. Postoperative image shown good alignment. Calcium sulfate filling the defect fully but the cement outside of bone defect between distal radius and ulna. Potential risk is irritating soft tissue cellulites.

5.2 Impact on fracture healing

Calcium sulphate, as a synthetic bone graft substitute, has demonstrated the capability to support fracture healing. All cases in this study showed callus by X-ray in 2 to 4 months. The average time of bone callus appearing was 2.9 months. Distal radioulnar joint had good alignment (Figure 6, 7, 8, 9).

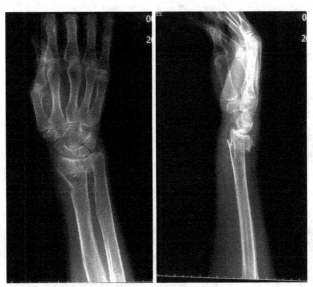

Fig. 6. Preoperative anteroposterior and lateral X-ray image demonstrated significant dorsal fracture displacement and distal collapse.

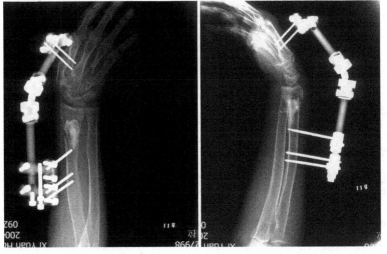

Fig. 7. Postoperative anteroposterior and lateral X-ray image shown good alignment. Calcium sulfate filling the defect fully was evident radiographically.

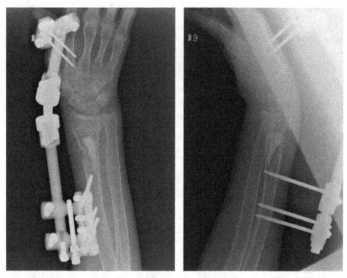

Fig. 8. Radiologic examination 4 weeks after surgery showed partial resorption of calcium sulphate.

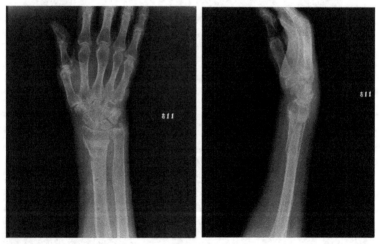

Fig. 9. At 8 weeks after surgery the calcium sulphate was absorbed completely and callus formation and fracture stability was demonstrated. The external fixator was removed.

In the majority of cases it seems that the appearance of callus and new bone were later than the time for material absorption, which means the callus appeared after the cement was absorbed. In this study we found 86% of the patients with calcium sulphate were absorbed within 2 months with the complete absorption at 3 months.

Borrelli[15] et al assessed the calcium sulfate cement had bending and torsional strength comparable with autogenous bone in treated bone defects cases. The authors also observed that calcium sulphate had adequate mechanical strength and believe that the absorption of calcium sulfate and bone callus formation in the implantation site is predictable and simultaneous. Therefore there should be reduced concern if the calcium sulphate is absorbed in 2 or 3 months after surgery if proper external fixation support is achieved.

6. Conclusions

It is recommended to use injection of calcium sulphate bone graft material in the treatment of comminuted distal radius fractures, especially in metaphyseal fracture defects. Minimally invasive approach causes reduced damage to the tissue, significantly decreasing the risk of infection and accelerating the bone healing. Overfilling or pressurizing the defect site should be avoided. There is the potential to cause a reaction if the bone graft material overspills into the soft tissue, in addition to potential articular cartilage damage if extravasation into the joint space occurs. Kelley and Borrelli reported that 3% to 7% of the site drainage and cellulitis are related to the product itself; such phenomenon requires further clinical investigation. In cases where sterile wound drainage occurs, changing dressings for a few days usually resolves the problem. Bacterial culture or giving prophylactic antibiotics are only needed if it is suspected that an infection is present.

Synthetic calcium sulphate bone cement is an ideal choice of bone graft substitute for stabilization and repair of comminuted distal radius fractures by minimally invasive technique and external fixation. The capability to support new bone formation is excellent and the material absorption is 100%. Calcium sulphate also has the advantage of being mouldable such that it can be shaped to fill gaps in bone, in addition to setting hard within a convenient time frame (approximately 10 minutes), combined with good mechanical strength. It can also be injected for minimally invasive surgery. Calcium sulphate is now being used as a carrier for local delivery and slow release of antibiotics, so it is a material with a huge potential clinical application. The use of calcium sulphate to treat distal radial fracture defects coupled with external fixation appears safe and efficacious, if the articular surface defect is larger than 0.5cm or the gap of bone cavities is less than 2.5cm.

7. References

[1] Song HP & Wang ZQ. (2005). Interference Factors in the Clinical Effects of Bone Allograft. *Chinese Journal of Bone Tumor and Bone Disease*, Vol.4, No.4, (2005), pp. 245-248. Chinese

[2] Sun SQ & Li BX. (2003). Diseases transmitted after allograft bone grafting. *Chinese Journal of Bone Tumor and Bone Disease*, Vol.2, No.6, (2003), pp. 333-335. Chinese

[3] Malinin TI & Brown MD. (1981). Bone Allografts in Spinal Surgery. *Clin Orthop Rel Res*, Vol.154, (1981), pp. 68-73

[4] Lane JM & Sandhu HS. (1987). Current approaches to experimental bone grafting. *Orthop Clin North Am*, Vol.18, (1987), pp. 213-25

[5] Yang DF et al. (2010). The causes and strategies for the postoperative shortening in distal radius fractures. *Zhongguo Gu Shang.* V23N8(2010), 581-584

[6] Kelly CM et al. (2001). The Use of a Surgical Grade Calcium Sulfate as a Bone Graft Substitute. *Clin Orthop*, Vol.382, (2001), pp. 42-50

[7] Joseph B et al. Treatment of Nonunions and Osseous Defects with Bone Graft and Calcium Sulfate. *Clin Orthop.* 2002, 411-pp: 245-254

[8] Zhang Y et al. (2008). Less invasive leverage reduction with external fixator supported and bone graft for treatment of unstable fractures of distal radius. *Zhongguo Xiu Fu Chong Jian Wai Ke Za Zhi.* 2008V22N3:314-7

[9] Capo JT et al. (2010). Treatment of extra-articular distal radial malunions with an intramedullary implant. *J Hand Surg Am.* 2010V35N6:892-9

[10] Bavonratanavech S et al. (2005). Distal radial fractures: Injectable calcium phosphate bone cement versus conventional treatment. *Chinese Journal of Orthopaedic Trauma,* Vol 7. Issue 4, (2005), pp. 368-374

[11] Lobenhoffer P et al. (2002). Use of an Injectable Calcium Phosphate Bone Cement in the Treatment of Tibial Plateau Fractures: A Prospective Study of Twenty-Six Cases with Twenty-Month Mean Follow-Up. *J. Orthop Trauma,* Vol.16, No.3, pp. 143-149

[12] Walsh WR et al. (2003). Response of a Calcium Sulfate Bone Graft Substitute in a Confined Cancellous Defect. *Clin. Orthop.* Vol.406, (2003), pp. 228-236

[13] Gitelis S et al. (2001). Use of a Calcium Sulfate Based bone Graft Substitute for Benign Bone Lesions. *Orthopedics,* Vol.2, (2001), pp. 162-166

[14] Borrelli J et al. (2002). Treatment of Nonunions and Osseous Defects with Bone Graft and Calcium Sulfate. *Clin Orthop,*Vol.411, (2002), pp. 245-254

[15] Xu N et al. (2006). The Use of MIIG115-bone graft substitute in the Reconstruction of the distal end of the radius Comminuted Fracture. *Orthopedic Biomechanics Materials and Clinical study,* Vol.3, No.2, (2006), pp. 22-24. Chinese

9

Treatment of Chronic Osteomyelitis Using Vancomycin-Impregnated Calcium Sulphate Cement

Deng Lei, Ma Zhanzhong, Yang Huaikuo, Xue Lei, Yang Gongbo
Orthopedic Department of Beijing XiYuan Hospital,
China Academy of Chinese Medical Science,
China

1. Introduction

In the treatment of chronic osteomyelitis, the common methods in primary stage are debriding, draining and lavaging, but the clinical outcomes are not always satisfactory. Autogenous bone grafting in a second stage procedure has been the gold standard for this type of treatment, but its quantity is limited. In addition the autogenous bone graft will be absorbed or become sequestrum if the inflammation control is not sufficient [1][2]. Allogeneic bone, although solving the problem of limited supply, is likely to cause or increase the immune response and infection [3][4]. The availability of antibiotic loaded polymethylmethacrylate (PMMA) bone cement, particularly the antibiotic bead chain, provides a new direction for the treatment of osteomyelitis. However, antibiotic impregnated bone cements are non-absorbing, can support a biofilm and become a foreign body and nidus for infection at the implant site. They must be removed in a further surgical procedure if bone graft implantation is required.

In recent years, surgeons have paid increasing attention to calcium sulphate and calcium phosphate bone cements because of their biocompatibility, they are biodegradable, injectable and can be impregnated with antibiotics or other therapeutics. These advantages are more attractive for their use in infection cases. This study is based on the routine primary treatment of infection, and applies vancomycin-impregnated calcium sulphate cement to fill the focus cavity in a second stage procedure. The clinical results were satisfactory. The case reports are as follows.

2. Materials and methods

2.1 Materials and patient selection

There were 20 cases of chronic osteomyelitis in the patient group, 18 males and 2 females. Aged from 16 to 60 years old, the mean age was 41 years old. Classifying the cases according to the focus site, 1 case was in iliac, 4 cases were in femur, 5 cases were in the lower tibia and 10 cases were in calcaneus. All 20 cases suffered traumatic injury and initially had internal fixation. Although these patients had anti-infective treatment regimen immediately after surgery, all developed chronic osteomyelitis. The time to presentation with osteomyelitis was a minimum of 6 months and a maximum of 25 years (femoral and calcaneal osteomyelitis recurrent attack) after the index procedure. All patients had routine anti-infective treatment in the primary stage procedure and later were treated with implantation of vancomycin-impregnated calcium sulphate cement (Stimulan Kit). The details of information are in the table below.

case	Focus site	Surgical method		Result of treatment
		I stage Primary treatment	II stage Further treatment Stimulan+vancomycin	
1	Calcaneus (right)	Debriding, draining	After debridement again, fill vancomycin-impregnated calcium sulphate cement into the focus site 5cc calcium sulphate cement + 0.8g vancomycin	Wound Closed in primary stage, drainage occurred one week after surgery, treated and healed by changing dressings
2	Calcaneus (right)	Debriding, antibiotics chain, draining	10cc calcium sulphate cement + 1.6g vancomycin	Healed
3	Calcaneus (left)	Debriding, draining	10cc calcium sulphate cement + 1.6g vancomycin	Healed
4	Calcaneus (left)	Debriding, draining, antibiotics chain	5cc calcium sulphate cement + 0.8g vancomycin	Healed
5	Calcaneus (left)	Debriding, antibiotics chain	5cc calcium sulphate cement + 0.8g vancomycin	Healed
6	Calcaneus (left)	Debriding, antibiotics chain	5cc calcium sulphate cement + 0.8g vancomycin	Healed
7	Calcaneus (left)	Debriding, antibiotics chain	5cc calcium sulphate cement + 0.8g vancomycin	Healed
8	Calcaneus (left)	Debriding, antibiotics chain	5cc calcium sulphate cement + 0.8g vancomycin	Healed
9	Calcaneus (left)	Debriding, antibiotics chain	5cc calcium sulphate cement + 0.8g vancomycin	Healed

case	Focus site	Surgical method		Result of treatment
		I stage Primary treatment	II stage Further treatment Stimulan+vancomycin	
10	Calcaneus (bilateral)	Debriding, antibiotics chain	15cc calcium sulphate cement + 2.4g vancomycin	Closed wound in the primary stage, drainage occurred one week after surgery, treated and healed by changing dressings
11	Iliac (right)	Debriding and simultaneous removal of internal fixation, draining, lavaging	After debridement again, focus site filled with vancomycin-impregnated calcium sulphate cement 25cc calcium sulphate cement + 4.0g vancomycin	Healed
12	Middle femur (right)	Debriding, draining, lavaging, antibiotics chain	After debriding again, focus site filled with vancomycin-impregnated calcium sulphate cement 30cc calcium sulphate cement + 4.8g vancomycin	Healed
13	Middle femur (right)	Draining, lavaging, antibiotics chain	After debriding again, focus site filled with vancomycin-impregnated calcium sulphate cement 20cc calcium sulphate cement + 3.2g vancomycin	Healed
14	Middle femur (right)	Draining, lavaging, antibiotics chain	After debriding again, focus site filled with vancomycin-impregnated calcium sulphate cement 20cc calcium sulphate cement + 3.2g vancomycin	Healed
15	Middle femur (left)	Debriding, draining, lavaging	After debriding again, focus site filled with vancomycin-impregnated calcium sulphate cement 20cc calcium sulphate cement + 3.2g vancomycin	Focus site filled with vancomycin-impregnated calcium sulphate cement into the focus site 2 times Eventually healed

case	Focus site	Surgical method		Result of treatment
		I stage Primary treatment	**II stage** Further treatment Stimulan+vancomycin	
16	Lower tibia (left)	Debriding, draining, lavaging, antibiotics bone cement	After debriding again, focus site filled with vancomycin-impregnated calcium sulphate cement 25cc calcium sulphate cement + 4.0g vancomycin	Drainage occurred 3 weeks after surgery, treated and healed by changing dressings
17	Lower tibia (right)	Debriding, draining, lavaging, antibiotics chain	After debriding again, focus site filled with vancomycin-impregnated calcium sulphate cement 20cc calcium sulphate cement + 3.2g vancomycin	Healed
18	Lower tibia (right)	Draining, lavaging, antibiotics chain	After debriding again, focus site filled with vancomycin-impregnated calcium sulphate cement 20cc calcium sulphate cement + 3.2g vancomycin	Healed
19	Lower tibia (right)	Draining, lavaging, antibiotics chain	After debriding again, focus site filled with vancomycin-impregnated calcium sulphate cement 30cc calcium sulphate cement + 4.8g vancomycin	Healed
20	Lower tibia (left)	Draining, lavaging, antibiotics chain	After debriding again, focus site filled with vancomycin-impregnated calcium sulphate cement 15cc calcium sulphate cement + 2.4g vancomycin	Healed

2.2 Methods for treatment

Primary stage treatment: Routine treatment of chronic osteomyelitis includes resection of soft tissue focus, removal of sequestrum, fenestration drainage of bone lesions (ilium, calcaneus), lavaging (tibia, femur) and polishing the surface of sclerotic bone with a burr. In addition to the methods above, for long bone with a closed marrow cavity, firstly add antibiotic bead chain or antibiotic bone cement as the anti-inflammatory transitional stage when drilling medullary cavity and lavage at the same time. The cement is then removed in the revision surgery 4 to 6 weeks later. The bacterial culture and sensitivity tests are carried out as routine preoperative examination before the surgery. Only 1 case of femoral osteomyelitis in this group was staphylococcus aureus positive, other cases were all negative.

Second stage treatment: 4-6 weeks after all the patients had primary routine treatment, and local infected sites had shown no irritation, pain or purulent exudates. Surgical sites were then filled with vancomycin-impregnated calcium sulphate cement and the wound closed immediately. The common dosage of antibiotics was 1g vancomycin in 5cc calcium sulphate cement. Depending on different sizes of the focus, the volume of calcium sulphate cement used ranged from 5cc- 30cc (case 1, 2). The author has found that the calcaneal osteomyelitis may have high recurrent risk due to the infected area having more cancellous bone. Therefore we pay more attention when performing second stage treatment. Before the second stage treatment is carried out, a negative bacteria culture must be achieved and second time debridement must be carried out before the use of the vancomycin-impregnated cement. In addition, the sclerotic bone needs to be trimmed and the sequestrum space needs to be debrided and cleaned completely. The infected cavities should be filled as tightly as possible without leaving dead space in order to maximize the treatment with antibiotics.

3. Result

Stitches were removed 3 weeks after surgery. 17 cases showed stage I wound healing. 2 cases in the calcaneus and 1 case in the tibia showed site drainage after surgery, but no purulent secretions were found and the bacterial cultures were negative. The wound gradually healed after changing dressings. No recurrences of infection or pathological fractures were found after 10 to 30 months follow-up. The antibiotic-impregnated cement was completely absorbed within 3 months and ossification in the bone defect was 100%. No systemic abnormal reactions were found.

4. Discussion

4.1

The treatment of chronic osteomyelitis has become a difficult problem in orthopaedics as it is difficult to eradicate. Due to the availability of new materials and methods, many new concepts and technologies have been developed for treatment of chronic osteomyelitis on the basis of regular treatment. The uses of non-absorbable antibiotic-impregnated bone cement and absorbable biological bone cement to treat the infection have been reported recently subsequent to routine antibiotics chains being used. Non-absorbable bone cement needs to be removed after the antibiotics has released and the local concentration of antibiotics released in soft tissue, bones and joints is lower than levels delivered by antibiotic-impregnated absorbable biological cement [5]. The commonly used antibiotics for impregnation today are Gentamycin, Kanamycin, Tobramycin, and Rifampin. Quinolones have also been reported such as Moxifloxacin [6]; the common drug carriers include medical grade calcium phosphate cement (CPC) [7] [8] [9], Hydroxyapatite [10] [11] and PMMA bone cement. However the reported use of vancomycin-impregnated calcium sulphate cement (CSC) is less common. In the application of antibiotic-impregnated biological cement, it is necessary to choose not only the effective antibiotics but also the carriers. The carriers must have same crystal structure in terms same size and shape in order to encourage the osteogenesis. If a carrier is absorbed too fast, it will decrease the function of osteoconductivity, while if a carrier is absorbed too slow, it will inhibit new bone formation. Pharmaceutical grade calcium sulphate cement, Stimulan Kit, is synthetically produced from high purity reagents. It has a physiologic pH and a higher purity compared to calcium sulphate prepared from gypsum rock. Stability and the absorption speed are close to new bone formation speed. So we believe that the calcium sulphate is an ideal antibiotic carrier. We used self-made vancomycin-impregnated calcium sulphate cement in all cases. 17 cases showed wound healing in first stage and the other 3 cases gradually healing after changing dressings.

Tomoyuki et al reported that the concentration level of antibiotics releasing in vancomycin-impregnated calcium sulphate cement was 50 times and 13 times that of PMMA bone cement at 1 and 2 weeks after use, which greatly enhanced the efficacy in local focus. Kyriaki et al carried out a comparison study of vancomycin-impregnated calcium sulphate cement and PMMA bone cement and reported that the concentration level of local antibiotics releasing in former was much higher than the latter. Many experimental studies have confirmed that the level of antibiotics released by vancomycin-impregnated calcium sulphate cement is higher than PMMA bone cement. In addition, vancomycin-impregnated calcium sulphate cement produces no heat of polymerization, is completely absorbed and releases all of the antibiotic load. It also will not affect the osteogenesis in focus site.

4.2

Complete primary first stage treatment is an essential step for antibiotics-impregnated calcium sulphate cement filling. Since systemic antibiotic treatment is less effective in the treatment of chronic osteomyelitis, focus site treatment become critical. The bacterial culture in chronic osteomyelitis is often gram negative, which is considered to be related to long term antibiotic use and low grade toxicity of the bacteria. In this study, all cases took secretion culture and drug susceptibility tests before and after surgery. Only one case in femoral focus cultured positive for staphylococcus aureus, the others were all clear. Treatment methods included debriding thoroughly, polishing the surface of sclerotic bone with a burr, and adequate drainage. One case of iliac bone and 10 cases of calcaneus osteomyelitis carried out debridement and drainage until the drain was clear, then filled the antibiotic-impregnated calcium sulphate cement; 5 cases of tibial and 4 cases of femoral osteomyelitis had debridement and catheter flushing first. At the same time the canal was drilled and filled with self-made antibiotics chain or antibiotic bone cement. On removing the chain or antibiotic bone cement surgical sites were filled with vancomycin-impregnated calcium sulfate cement when lavaging fluid is clean after 4-6 weeks. After use of antibiotics chain, a drainage strip was placed. Although some antibiotic will be lost through the drain, a higher rate of wound healing was evident. Yang Xingguang [12] et al also reported that the drainage or lavage may be reduce the concentration of antibiotics, but it is important for the healing of soft tissue.

4.3

The main disadvantage for using PMMA bone cement is that it will become a foreign body after drug release. The authors found that bone cement, as a drug carrier, had not only a limited drug release, but was also associated with necrosis between the surface of cement and the surrounding tissue. It confirms the poor compatibility of bone cement in inflammatory tissue or it may be related with the elevated temperature effects during polymerization. It should therefore be removed. Some research has also confirmed adhesion of bacteria on the bone cement surface after using the antibiotic chain, speculating that this is one of the factors of recurrence of inflammation. As antibiotics-impregnated calcium sulphate cement is absorbable and demonstrates simultaneous absorption and osteogenesis, it will not result in necrosis adjacent to the material and will eliminate the focus infection. The X-ray follow up also demonstrated and confirmed the absorption of calcium sulphate cement was matched with the speed of osteogenesis. The X-rays were taken in all cases and osteogenesis was found in all at 3 to 4 weeks after surgery with partial absorption of the calcium sulphate. The calcium sulphate cement was fully absorbed after 3 months and the local new bone formed well.

4.4

The clinical efficacy of absorbable bone cement, as a drug carrier, will be influenced by the setting time, strength, the level of concentration, the antibiotic elution rate and the porosity of the set cement. In order to ensure the releasing concentration of vancomycin did not affect the calcium sulfate bone cement's strength after solidification in this study, the ratio of vancomycin and cement was 0.8g vancomycin/5cc calcium sulphate. The setting time and strength of calcium sulphate did not change in the surgery. Osamu's tests showed that when using PMMA as the antibiotic carrier, the effective drug release is not as high as the absorbable antibiotic-impregnated cement. Michal et al used injectable antibiotic-impregnated cement to treat chronic osteomyelitis, the preliminary tests also showing positive results.

The authors believe that vancomycin-impregnated calcium sulfate cement performs the function of filling bone voids and dead space and maintaining effective release of antibiotics. The local concentration of antibiotics releasing in calcium sulphate is higher than observed with antibiotic loaded PMMA bead chains or antibiotic loaded PMMA bone cement, and can be many times the minimum inhibitory concentration (MIC) for the involved pathogen. Treatment of chronic osteomyelitis using self-made vancomycin-impregnated calcium sulfate cement has achieved a satisfactory therapeutic effect. Therefore the authors recommend it as a method to treat chronic osteomyelitis.

5. Case accessories

Case 1: Male, 40 years old. Patient sustained left distal tibia and fibula fractures (Pilon fracture) caused by traffic accident. Infection appeared after wire fixation and developed osteomyelitis. Infection invaded to the ankle joint and the talus just three months after the first operation. Although patient had kept the wound clean, and changed dressing, the wound remained unhealed. The patient was transferred to our unit 8 months after initial trauma. Patient was twice cleared and underwent debridement. Antibiotic PMMA bone cement was used to fill the bone marrow cavity of tibia and ankle, with a drain present. 6 weeks later, the bone cement was removed and the void filled with self-made vancomycin-impregnated calcium sulfate cement. The osteomyelitis of the tibia and talus was eradicated 6 weeks after using vancomycin-impregnated calcium sulfate cement. The calcium sulfate cement began to be absorbed, and callus began to grow at 10 weeks (Fig. 1, 2).

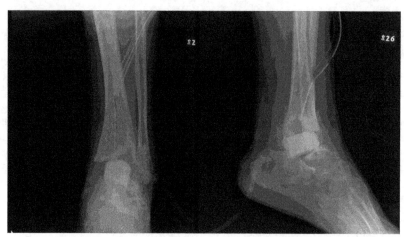

Fig. 1. After debridement, antibiotics bone cement was implanted and catheter drainage was placed.

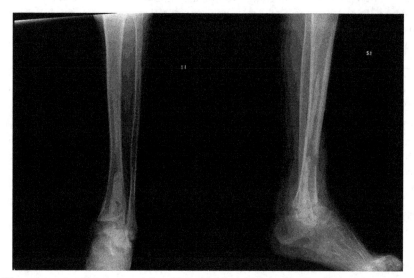

Fig. 2. The calcium sulfate cement began to be absorbed, and callus began to grow at 10 weeks.

Case 2: Female, 50 years old. Patient suffered chronic osteomyelitis after calcaneus fracture surgery. Patient underwent debridement treatment and initial fixation plates were removed. Antibiotic loaded PMMA bone cement was implanted in the cavity. Patient underwent secondry debridement treatment 8 weeks later and vancomycin-impregnated calcium sulphate cement was placed. The wound healed three weeks later and the stitches were removed. CT follow up show vancomycin-impregnated calcium sulphate cement was partially absorbed and callus appeared at the fracture defect two months after placing the vancomycin-impregnated calcium sulphate cement.

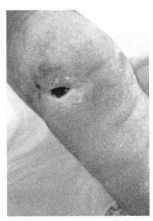

Fig. 3. Infection and persistent sinus occurred after calcaneus fracture surgery and the wound was not healed. The patient was transferred to our unit and debridement treatment was given and antibiotic loaded PMMA cement chain was placed until the sinus was clean, free of leakage with no bacterial growth.

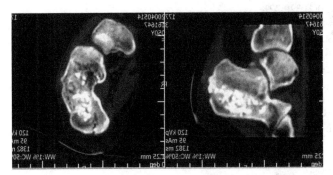

Fig. 4. Patient had secondary surgery and antibiotics-impregnated calcium sulphate cement was placed. CT showed that the antibiotics-impregnated calcium sulphate cement in the calcaneus was partially absorbed.

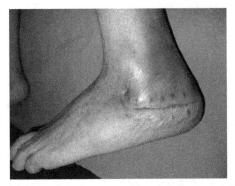

Fig. 5. The wound healed fully and patient was able to perform weight-bearing exercises.

6. References

[1] Malinin TL & Brown MD. (1981). Bone allografts in spinalo surgery. Clin. Orthop, 1981, 154: 68-73

[2] Lane JM & Sandhu HS. (1987). Cuurrent approaches to experimental bone grafting. Orthop Clin North Am, 1987, 18:213-25

[3] Song HP & Wang Zh Q. (2005). The interference factors of clinical results with allogeneic bone graft. Chinese Journal of Bone Tumor and Bone Disease, 2005, 4:245-248

[4] Sun Sh Q & Li BX. (2003). Disease Transmission of allogeneic bone graft. Chinese Journal of Bone Tumor and Bone Disease，2003，2:333-335

[5] Michal YK, et al. (2007). Gentamicin extended release from an injectable polymeric implants Journal of Controlled Release, 2007, 117:90-96

[6] Kyriaki K, et al.(2006). Comparative elution of moxifloxacin from Norian skeletal repair system and acrylic bone cement; an in vitro study. International Journal of Antimicrobial Agents. 2006, 28:217-220

[7] Tomoyuki S MD, et al.(2005). In Vitro Elution of Vancomycin from Calcium Phosphate Cement. The Journal of Arthroplasty, 2005, 20(2): 1055-1059

[8] Takahiro Niikura, et al.(2007). Vancomycin-impreganted Calcium Phosphate Cement for Methicillinresistant Staphylococcus aureus Femoral Osteomyelitis Orthopedics, 2007, 30(4):320-321

[9] Anna D, et al.(2005). The effect of processing on the structural characteristics of vancomycin-loaded amorphous calcium phosphate matrices. Biomaterials, 2005, 26: 4486-4494

[10] Osamu Kisanuki et al. (2007). Experimental study of calcium phosphate cement impregnated with dideoxy-kanamycin. B J Orthop. Sci, 2007, 12:281-288

[11] Geng Sh R, et al (1995). The study and using of artificial bone with calcium hydroxyapatite glass ceramic. Chinese journal of bone and joint injury, 1995,10 (6): 323-361

[12] Yang XG, et al. (2004). Self-solidifying calcium phosphate artificial bone with Septopal chain to treat traumatic osteomyelitis. Orthopedic Journal of China. 2004, 12 (15): 1146-1148

10

Spinal Fusion with Methylmethacrylate Cage

Majid Reza Farrokhi and Golnaz Yadollahi Khales

Shiraz Neurosciences Research Center, Shiraz University of Medical Sciences, Shiraz, Iran

1. Introduction

A brief history of anterior cervical decompression and fusion (ACDF) surgery is useful. The first reports on ventral approaches to cervical disc pathology appeared in the 1950s. Two most common methods for ACDF were described by Robinson and Smith in 1955 (1) and Cloward in 1958 (2). Robinson and Smith described a surgical procedure for removing cervical disc material in which a rectangular bone graft, obtained from the iliac crest, was replaced to allow a cervical fusion to develop. In Cloward's method, discectomy was performed by a dowel technique. Although numerous modifications have been made to this procedure since the 1950s, a great majority of spine surgeons currently use either the Cloward or the Robinson and Smith's technique. Now, this technique is used in special circumstances. Marked motor deficit or agonizing intractable radicular pain with an appropriate disc imaging is a Principal indication for expedient intervention in root syndromes. Additionally, a myelopathic picture from soft central sequestra is an ordinarily reason for prompt surgery. Chronic persistent brachialgia with nerve root symptoms appropriate to the findings obtained from imaging warrants surgical treatment. Surgery is also indicated if there is a tumor or infection that compresses the cord (3).

1.1 History of spinal fusion

In 1911, Albee (4) and Hibbs (5) used spinal fusion for stabilization. Although it was performed to prevent progressive spinal deformity in patients with Pott's disease, the procedure was later used to manage scoliosis and traumatic fractures. Hibbs' method, which was most frequently used, comprised harvesting an autologous bone graft from the laminae and overlaying the bone dorsally. Despite later improvements in this technique, the rate of pseudarthrosis especially in scoliosis remained unacceptably high (6). Robinson and Smith (1) described their technique in 1955 and Cloward (2) described his cervical fusion technique in 1958.

1.2 Biology of spine fusion

Each year, more than 185,000 spinal arthrodeses are performed in the United States that most of them are posterolateral lumbar intertransverse process fusions (7). There should be several factors working together to obtain a successful fusion including local environment of fusion, systemic factors, and possible use of fusion enhancers.

2. Graft properties

Choosing graft material has profound implications for success or failure of an arthrodesis. The ideal graft is osteogenic, osteoinductive, and osteoconductive.

2.1 Osteoinduction

Osteoinduction is the stimulation of multipotential stem cells for differentiation into functioning osteogenic cells. This is mediated by growth factors in bone matrix itself. Both autogenous and allograft bone are osteoinductive (8).

2.2 Osteogenicity

Osteogenicity refers to the presence of viable osteogenic cells, either predetermined or inducible, within the graft. Only fresh autologous bone and bone marrow are osteogenic (9).

2.3 Osteoconduction

Osteoconductivity refers to a material's capacity to foster neovascularization and infiltration by osteogenic precursor cells via creeping substitution. It occurs on the scaffold provided by bone graft matrix.

2.4 Connectivity

Connectivity is the ability of an osteoconductive graft material to be connected to the local bone. This is determined by the surface area available for incorporation into the fusion mass.

3. Graft material

3.1 Autograft

Autogenous bone from iliac crest is the gold standard graft material. Historically, it has been the most successful graft source in spinal fusion. Cancellous autograft has the requisite matrix proteins, mineral, and collagen for the ideals of osteoinductivity, osteogenicity, and osteoconductivity. Nevertheless, there are significant drawbacks to autograft including procurement morbidity, limited availability, and increased operative time (10).

3.2 Allograft

The desire to avoid donor site morbidity led to increased use of allograft bone in spine surgery. Advances in procurement, sterilization, preparation, and storage made it practical. Although it was widely used in the spine surgery, there are still concerns regarding fusion rates and disease transmission. Allograft is not osteogenic because there is no surviving cell in the graft. Some osteoinductive potential of allograft is lost for processing and storage requirements of allograft. Although allograft is generally performed well in both cervical and lumbar interbody fusions in which the graft is subject to compression, the results of posterolateral lumbar environment with primarily tensile forces are not favorable. This has led many surgeons to use allograft as an autograft (11). However, there are some complications such as graft collapse, graft expulsion, graft site pain and infection, pseudarthrosis, spinal deformity, and poor fusion rate (12). The low stabilizing effect of bone grafts often requires further stabilization with anterior plates (13).

3.3 Xenograft

Taking bone graft from other species has been reported in the orthopedic literature (14). Despite processes of xenografts, they remain immunogenic and provoke a host response. The graft may be encapsulated with resultant blockade to be revascularized (15).

4. Bone substitutes

Because of these drawbacks in both autograft and allograft tissues, synthetic alternatives have been a very active area of research for the past 20 years. Nevertheless, only 10% of the 2.2 million bone graft procedures worldwide involve synthetics for the perceived inferiority to native autograft and allograft. Drawbacks of many synthetics include poor resorbability, inclusion of animal or marine-derived components, variable handling characteristics, limited availability, and increased cost (16).

4.1 Ceramics

Tricalcium phosphate $(Ca_3(PO_4)_2)$ ceramics including hydroxyapatite (HA) and tricalcium phosphate (TCP) have been widely used in orthopedic and spine surgery (17). These osteoconductive, biodegradable materials are compatible with the remodeling of bone necessary to achieve optimal strength. Other non-resorbable materials remain in the fusion mass, leave permanent stress risers and prolong strength deficiencies. Synthetics should have several properties to be a useful graft material. $Ca_3(PO_4)_2$ ceramics are compatible with local tissues, remain chemically stable in body fluids, and should be able to withstand sterilization. (18) Furthermore, they should be available in different shapes and size, be cost-effective, and have reliable quality control. These ceramics have been widely used in dentistry and maxillofacial surgery, (19) as well as in animal models (20). They are also used in humans and may be prepared as either compact or porous materials. Greater crystallinity and density of compact forms results in greater strength and resistance to dissolution in *vivo*. However, more porous versions which approximate the interconnectivity of cancellous bone enhance bone ingrowth at the expense of more rapid degradation. Natural coral is successfully used for augmentation or even replacement autograft (21). The calcium carbonate $(CaCO_3)$ in coral is hydrothermally converted to $Ca_3(PO_4)_2$. The structural geometry of coral is similar to cancellous bone that makes it highly osteoconductive and connective.

5. Non injectable ceramics

Synthetic ceramics are osteoconductive but do not intrinsically possess any osteoinductive potential. The most common ceramics in current use are hydroxyapatite $[Ca_{10}(PO_4)_6(OH)_2]$, tricalcium phosphate $[Ca_3(PO_4)_2]$, calcium sulfate dihydrate $[CaSO_4 \cdot 2H_2O]$, and combinations of that. In spite of exhibiting different chemical properties from tissue grafts, ceramics provide off-the-shelf availability of consistently high-quality synthetic materials with no biologic hazards. After incorporation, the strength of the repaired defect site is comparable to that of cancellous bone. Therefore, ceramics can be used as an alternative or an addition to either cancellous autograft or allograft, as cancellous bone void filler, bone graft extender, or in sites where compression is in a dominant mode of mechanical loading (22).

5.1 Rapidly resorbing ceramics

Scaffolds of tricalcium phosphate have two forms including α and β that are formulated at 1200 °C and 800°C, respectively (23). These forms have different crystalline structures but the same elemental and stoichiometric characteristics.

5.2 Intermediate resorbing ceramics

5.2.1 β- Tricalcium phosphate

An ultraporous β-tricalcium phosphate (β-TCP) formulation, engineered using nanoparticle technology, has porosity comparable to natural cancellous bone (24).

5.3 Slowly resorbing ceramics

Hydroxyapatite is another ceramic that is readily available, but is associated with extremely slow remodeling. Slowly resorbing or nonresorbing material can interfere with remodeling and be the nidus of a mechanical stress point. Slow resorption and brittleness of hydroxyapatite make it less ideal for clinical use. Therefore, hydroxyapatite is often used in modified forms, for example, combining it with calcium carbonate to speed the rate of resorption (25).

6. Injectable ceramics (calcium phosphate cement)

In contrast to preformed solid constructs of calcium phosphate, so formed outside the body by manufacturing methods and subsequently placed by surgical intervention, liquid components can be injected directly into a bone defect site. This can then set into solid, defect filling, cement-like mass of calcium phosphate. Then it transforms slowly into bone in 3 to 4 years (26).The transformation of liquid components into a solid mass of calcium phosphate is achieved by well-known chemical reactions with a low-temperature exotherm. The resulting bone filler has a biologic response and compressive strength similar to cancellous bone (27) and promises some clinical applications such as adjunct treatment of vertebral body compression fractures and possibly the augmentation of pedicle screw fixation.

7. Nonbiologic osteoconductive substrates

Advantages of nonbiologic osteoconductive substrates include absolute control of final structure, no immunogenicity, and excellent biocompatibility (28). Some examples are degradable polymers, bioactive glasses, and porous metals such as tantalum.

8. Spinal implants: Rigid versus dynamic

Spinal implants can be described as rigid, dynamic, or hybrid. Dynamic implants provide some subsidence between segments. An advantage of a dynamic implant is that it can offset stress at the implant-bone interface and therefore does not provide stress shielding of the bone graft. The purpose of a rigid construct is to immobilize completely the spine. This is rarely achieved because of the properties of bone. Movement in a rigid system often increases with time through the weakening of the implant-bone interface. Repetitive movement under sufficient stress will eventually lead to failure at the interface, unless bony fusion first occurs. The goal of rigid fixation is only to hold long enough for bony fusion to take place. The purpose of a dynamic construct is to provide intersegmental subsidence.

9. Stainless steel

Stainless steel implants are iron and carbon-based alloys. Initial trials of stainless steels, as an implant, showed that preventing corrosion by aiding resistance to chloride degradation was insufficient (29).

10. Titanium-based alloys

Titanium-based alloys are currently the most commonly used alloys for bioimplantation. Titanium-based alloys are advantageous for several reasons. They have both high strength and fatigue resistance. Titanium based alloys also decrease stiffness compared to stainless steel. The reduction in the stiffness facilitates transfer of the stress at the bone-implant interfaces with alloy and can minimize bone resorption. Titanium-based alloys have higher fatigue strength compared to stainless steel. However, titanium alloys are vulnerable to any surface flaws. Any scratch or notch can rapidly accelerate the fatigue failure process. Titanium alloys also lack any known immunogenicity (30).

11. Interbody cages

A variety of prosthetic interbody cages are now available for use in the cervical spine, both for disc space arthrodesis and to bridge the larger voids created by single or multilevel corpectomy. Current devices are fabricated either from titanium alloy or polymer. Interbody cages are intended to confer immediate structural integrity to the ventral spine. Although some surgeons have placed them as naked implants, (31) more typically they are hollow, porous implants employed as carriers for osteoinductive or osteoconductive materials for securing long-term stability through biologic integration with the recipient spine. Some of their shortcomings are migration, subsidence, stenotic myelopathy, foreign body reactions and nonunion (32). Cages can also lead to computed tomography (CT) artifacts by obscuring interbody fusion.

12. Polyetheretherketone (PEEK)

PEEK cages have recently been used in cervical surgery. PEEK is polyetheretherketone, a semi-crystal polyaromatic linear polymer (33). PEEK is a non-absorbable biopolymer that has been used in a variety of industries including medical devices. The PEEK cages are biocompatible, radiolucent, and have modulus of elasticity similar to the bone. This distinguishing feature seems to be able to prevent cage subsidence induced by metallic cages (34). In an in vitro biomechanical study, the stiffness of the PEEK cage was statistically higher than that of the normal motion segment in flexion. Volume-related stiffness of the PEEK cage was higher than that of iliac bone in all directions. In addition to the fact that the

PEEK cage is radiolucent and does not produce artifacts on radiographs or CT scans, it is easy to evaluate fusion status on X-ray films. It also induces cell attachment and fibroblast proliferation and increases the protein content of the osteoblasts (35). There was no foreign body reaction in our series (36).

13. Bioabsorbable cages

Synthetic, absorbable, polymeric devices represent a new class of materials for achieving interbody fusion in the spine. The materials are typically radiolucent, have a low modulus of elasticity similar to that of bone, and will be completely absorbed over time (from 6 weeks to 6 years). Their radiolucent nature improves image assessment of fusion healing, and their time-engineered resorption characteristics allow controlled dynamization in interbody and plate applications. However, their degradation elicits a mild inflammatory response and may in more severe cases cause osteolysis and/or sterile sinus drainage. Furthermore, an absorbable device would not be able to continue supporting the disc space in a pseudarthrosis. The clinical use of absorbable cervical spine cages made of 40% poly (N-vinylpyrrolidone comethylmethacrylate), 50% polyamide fibers and 10% calcium gluconate was first reported in 1989 with early positive results. However, subsequent studies have reported low fusion rates, a high incidence of device migration, lack of incorporation into the surrounding bone, and questionable resorption. More recently, absorbable devices made from 70:30 poly (L-lactide:D, Llactide) copolymer (PLDLA) have been investigated for spinal fusion (37).

14. Biocompatibility

All surgical procedures are associated with a disruption of normal anatomic tissue planes which results in an accumulation of exudative fluid, fibrin, platelets, and polymorphonuclear leukocytes. 3 to 5 days postsurgery, macrophages accumulate and remove the surgical debris. 10 days after surgery, the macrophages are no longer present and lymphocytes predominate. It is followed by fibroblasts which complete the cellular phase of healing. Ceramic implants are very biocompatible since the cellular response to wound healing is not significantly altered. However, immune system is activated in the presence of a metal implant. For most surgical constructs, stainless steel implants are sufficiently nonreactive to permit bone fusion before the deleterious consequences of the normal inflammatory response such as severe pain or loosening. Metal allergy is widely prevalent and well recognized. Metal ions alone will not stimulate the immune system. Linked with proteins, metals such as cobalt, chromium, and especially nickel are immunogenic. Osteolysis or periprosthetic bone loss may occur at an implant site. Structural remodeling of surrounding bone occurs in response to stress shielding. This bone destruction can lead to possible failure of the implant and loosening (38).

15. History of bone cement

The story of modern cements began with Otto Röhm's invention of polymethyl methacrylate (PMMA), a solid material with good biocompatibility that was named plexiglass, in the early 20th century.

In 1943, polymerisation of PMMA became possible at room temperature. PMMA was used clinically for the first time in plastic surgery in the 1940s to close gaps in the skull. Comprehensive clinical tests of compatible bone cements with body were conducted before using them in surgery. The excellent tissue compatibility of PMMA allowed the use of bone cements for anchorage of head prostheses in the 1950s. In 1954, Idelberger (39) used PMMA to fill spinal defects.

In the 1960s, Charnley (40) began using bone cement in numerous patients for the fixation of both the femur and acetabulum. Later researchers came up with the idea of adding an antibiotic to cement to decrease the incidence of infection.

16. Synthetic polymers

Synthetic polymer production is a field of implant technology that is rapidly expanding. Polymers, commonly known as plastics, are typically very large molecules made from a large number of individual subunits called monomers. Polymers are chemical compounds formed by combining these smaller, repeating structural units. The subunits repeat in various patterns following principles similar to those of molecular biology. The covalent bonds in polymers have a Hexed length. The complex folding of polymers is created by weak hydrogen bond cross-links that permit unfolding and elongation. The two most commonly used polymers are PMMA and ultra-high molecular weight polyethylene (UHMWPE).Polymer can be made less flexible by stiffening the backbone molecular chain and increasing the cross-links. Numerous other properties can be influenced by chemical changes including density, crystallization, solubility, thermal stability, and strength. Ultra-high molecular weight polyethylene has been extensively used in artificial joints for its favorable surface wear and creep properties. In spine surgery, PMMA has been extensively used because it causes additional polymerization when the powder and liquid are mixed. The intermediate phase of polymerization yields a doughy material that can be worked and shaped into complex defects before it hardens. PMMA has many molecular and macroscopic defects that contribute to its characteristically weak tensile strength. These defects originate in the powder phase that consists of microspheres. The microspheres are bound together as the methylmethacrylate (MMA) monomer (liquid phase) polymerizes into a matrix that incorporates the microspheres. The juncture between the powder phase microspheres and the liquid phase remains relatively weak even after hardening. Additionally, the polymer chains have a few cross-links. In light of these reasons, the polymerized PMMA has a low tensile strength. The advantages of bone cement (acrylic polymer) over bone grafts and other cages are long-term clinical experience, high immediate stability, low donor site morbidity (41), low subsidence rate (42), and only mild inflammatory reactions. Nevertheless, bone cement is associated with polymerization heat, cytotoxicity, and false bony fusion (43).

17. Bone cement components

Two primary components of bone cements are a powder consisting of copolymers based on the substance PMMA, and a liquid monomer, MMA. These two components are mixed at an approximate ratio of 2:1 to form PMMA cement. Exposure to light or high temperatures can cause premature polymerization of the liquid component. Therefore, hydroquinone is added as a stabiliser or inhibitor to prevent premature polymerization. A starter, di-benzoyl peroxide (BPO), is added to the powder and an initiator, mostly N-dimethyl-p-toluidine (DmpT), is added to the liquid to encourage the polymer and monomer to polymerise at room temperature (cold curing cement). A contrast agent is added to make the cement radiopaque. Commercially available cements use either zirconium dioxide (ZrO_2) or barium sulphate ($BaSO_4$). Zirconium dioxide is one hundred times less soluble than barium sulphate with less effect on the mechanical properties of cement.

Chlorophyll is added to Biomet Europe cements, the color makes the cement more easily visible in the operating room, especially during revision procedures. The powder component in our antibiotic-loaded bone cement additionally contains an antibiotic (such as gentamicin) or a combination of antibiotics (such as gentamicin and clindamycin).

17.1 Kinds of bone cement

Bone cements may be divided into two kinds including low and high viscosity.

17.2 Low viscosity

These cements have a long-lasting liquid or mixing phase which causes a short working phase. Consequently, the application of low viscosity cements requires strict adherence to application times.

17.3 High viscosity

These cements have a short mixing phase and lose their stickiness quickly. They cause a longer working phase which gives the surgeon more time to apply them.

18. Polymerization

When the polymer powder and monomer liquid are mixed together, the polymerization process begins. The polymerization process can be divided into four different phases: mixing, waiting, application and setting.

18.1 Mixing phase

In the mixing phase, the cement should be mixed homogeneously to minimize the number of pores. Vacuum mixing is shown to reduce the porosity of the cement and to increase its mechanical strength.

18.2 Waiting phase

During this phase, the cements achieve a suitable viscosity for delivery of bone cement. The cement is still sticky dough in this phase.

18.3 Working phase

The working phase is a period during which the cement and the implant can be introduced. The cement should not be sticky and its viscosity should be suitable for application. If viscosity is very low, the cement may not be able to withstand the bleeding pressure and prevent blood from entering the cement (44).

18.4 Hardening phase

The cement hardens and sets completely during this phase. Cement temperature, the operation room temperature as well as the body temperature all influence hardening phase.

19. New acrylic cage

This acrylic cage is composed of PMMA and methacrylate and designed based on an experimental ring-to-cylinder (45). The cage has a curved, round plate adjustable to the upper endplate of the cervical disc space. The cages have a long internal cross-section of 14mm and a height of 5mm. The acrylic cage could be filled with 1 to 1.5 mL bone graft to be inserted into the disc space (fig.1). The acrylic cage showed significantly better distraction, higher biomechanical stiffness due to biomechanical properties of the acrylate polymer and cage design, lower range of motion in bending, and an early bony interbody fusion without major foreign body reaction compared to bone grafts (fig. 2, 3). Subsidence is less frequent within bone cement than with titanium or peek cages. It is explained by larger graft surface and better restoration of lordosis with acrylic cage than bone grafts and progressive interbody fusion (46). Furthermore, it has fewer CT artifacts, no bone cement toxicity or no heat effects, but it possibly reduces some of the long-term complications of other cages.

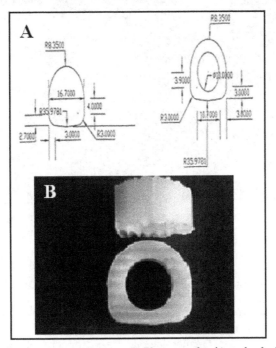

Fig. 1. A: Schematic drawing of acrylic cage. B: Photograph of interbody fusion cage designed to match the shape of cervical disc.

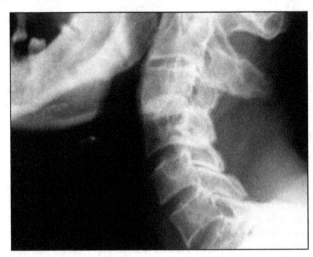

Fig. 2. Anterior cervical decompression and fusion (ACDF) with Acrylic cage at C3-C4 level extension view.

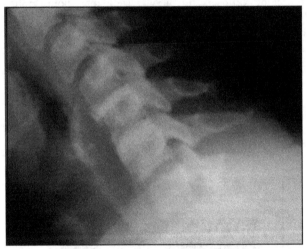

Fig. 3. Anterior cervical decompression and fusion (ACDF) with Acrylic cage at C4-C5 level FLx. vertebral.

20. References

[1] Robinson RA, Smith GW. Anterolateral cervical disc removal and interbody fusion for cervical disc syndrome. Bull john Hopkins Hasp1955; 95(1):223-224.
[2] Cloward RB. The anterior approach for removal of ruptured cervical disks. J Neurosurg 1958;15(6):602-17.
[3] Verbiest H, Paz y Geuse HD. Anterolateral surgery for cervical spondylosis in cases of myelopathy or nerve compression. J Neurosurg. 1966 ;25(6):611-22.

[4] Albee FH. Transplantation of a portion of the tibia into the spine for Pott's disease: a preliminary report 1911. Clin Orthop Relat Res 2007;460:14-6.

[5] Hibbs RA. An operation for progressive spinal deformities. Clin Orthop Relat Res 2007;460:17-20.

[6] Cloward HB. The anterior approach for removal of ruptured cervical disks. J Neurosurg Spine 2007;6(5):496-511

[7] Boden S. Overview of the biology of lumbar spine fusion and principles for selecting a bone graft substitute. Spine 2002; 27(16 suppl 1):S26-S31.

[8] Urist MR. Bone formation by autoinduction. Clin Orthop Relat Res 2002 ;(395):4-10.

[9] Urist MR, Silverman BF, Büring K, et al. The bone induction principle. Clin Orthop Relat Res 1967;53:243-83.

[10] Laurie SW, Kaban LB, Mulliken JB, et al. Donor site morbidity after harvesting rib and iliac bone. Plast Reconstr Surg 1984;73(6):933-8.

[11] Friedlander G.Current concepts review: bone banking. j Bone joint Surg 1966;48:915-923.

[12] Sawin PD, Traynelis VC, Menezes AH. A comparative analysis of fusion rates and donor-site morbidity of ontogenetic rib and iliac crest bone graft in posterior cervical fusion. J Neurosurg 1998;88: 255–265.

[13] Geisler FH, Caspar W, Pitzent T. Reoperation in patients after anterior cervical plate stabilization in degenerative disease. Spine (Phila Pa 1976). 1998 Apr 15;23(8):911-20.

[14] Prolo DJ, Rodrigo JJ. Contemporary bone graft physiology and surgery. Clin Orthop Relat Res 1985;(200):322-42.

[15] Harmon PH. Processed heterologous bone implants (Boplant, Squibb) as grafts in surgery. Acta Orthop Scand 1964;35:98-116.

[16] Lewandrowski KU, Gresser JO, Wise OL, et al. Bioresorbable bone graft substitutes of different osteoconductivities: a histologic evaluation of osteointegration of poly(propylene glycol-co-fumaric acid)-based cement implants in rats. Biomaterials. 2000 Apr;21(8):757-64.

[17] Bucholz R, Carlton A, Holmes R. Hydroxyapatite and tricalcium phosphate bone graft substitutes. Orthop Clin North Am. 1987 Apr;18(2):323-34.

[18] Flatley T, Lynch K, Benson M. Tissue response to implants of calcium phosphate ceramic in the rabbit spine. Clin Orthop Relat Res 1983;(179):246-52.

[19] Coviello J, Brilliant J. A preliminary study on the use of tricalcium phosphate as an apical barrier. J Endod 1979;5(1):6-13.

[20] Holmes R. Bone regeneration within a coralline hydroxyapatite implant. Plast Reconstr Surg 1979;63(5):626-33.

[21] Guillemin G, Meunier A, Dallant P, et al. Comparison of coral resorption and bone apposition with two natural corals of different porosities. J Biomed Mater Res 1989;23(7):765-79.

[22] Gazdag AR, Lane JM, Glaser D, et al. Alternatives to autogenous bone graft: efficacy and indications. J Am Acad Orthop Surg1955: 3(1):1-8.

[23] Cazeau C, Doursounian L, Touzard RC. Use of ceramics of calcum triphosphate in the repair of tibial plateau fractures: a series of 20 cases. European Journal of Orthopaedic Surgery & Traumatology 1999; 9 (3):171-174.

[24] Kon E, Muraglia A, Corsi A, et al. Autologous bone marrow stromal cells loaded onto porous hydroxyapatite ceramic accelerate bone repair in critical-size defects of sheep long bones. J Biomed Mater Res 2000;49(3):328-37.

[25] Fleming JE Jr, Cornell CN, Muschier GF. Bone cells and matrices in orthopedic tissue engineering. Orthop Clin North Am 2000;31(3):357-74.

[26] Sanchez-Sotelo J, Munuera L, Madero R. Treatment of fractures of the distal radius with a remodellable bone cement: a prospective, randomised study using Norian SRS. J Bone Joint Surg Br 2000;82(6):856-63.

[27] Constantz BR, Ison IC, Fulmer MT, et al. Skeletal repair by *in situ* formation of the mineral phase of bone. Science 1995;267(5205):1796-9.

[28] Cornell CN. Osteoconductive materials and their role as substitutes for autogenous bone grafts. Orthop Clin North Am 1999;30(4):591-8.

[29] Rae T. The toxicity of metals used in orthopaedic prosthesis. An experimental study using cultured human synovial fibroblasts. J Bone Joint Surg Br 1981;63-B(3):435-40.

[30] Jacobs JJ, Gilbert JL, Urban RM. Corrosion of metal orthopaedic implants. J Bone Joint Surg Am 1998;80(2):268-82.

[31] Lange M, Philipp A, Fink U, et al. Anterior cervical spine fusion using RABEA-Titan-Cages avoiding iliac crest spongiosa: first experiences and results. Neurol Neurochir Pol 2000;34(6 Suppl):64-9.

[32] Majd ME, Vadhva M, Hott RT. Anterior cervical reconstruction using titanium mesh cages with anterior plating. Spine (Phila Pa 1976). 1999 Aug 1;24(15):1604-10.

[33] Cho DY, Liau WR, Lee WY, et al. Preliminary experience using a polyetheretherketone (PEEK) cage in the treatment of cervical disc disease. Neurosurg.2002: 51(6):1343-50.

[34] Jen-Chung Liao, Chi-Chien Niu,Wen-Jer Chen, et al. Polyetheretherketone (PEEK) cage filled with cancellous allograft in anterior cervical discectomy and fusion. Int Orthop 2008; 32(5):643-8.

[35]. Petillo O, Peluso G, Ambrosio L, et al. In vivo induction of macrophage Ia antigen (MHC class II) expression by biomedical polymers in the cage implant system. J Biomed Mater Res1994; 28(5):635-46.

[36] Kahraman s, Daneyemez m, Kayali h, et al. Polyetheretherketone(Peek) Cages For Cervical Interbody Replacement:Clinical Experience. Turkish Neurosurgery 2006;16(3) 120-123.

[37] Slivka MA, Spenciner DB, Seim HB , et al. High Rate of Fusion in Sheep Cervical Spines Following Anterior Interbody Surgery With Absorbable and Nonabsorbable Implant Devices. Spine (Phila Pa 1976). 2006 Nov 15;31(24):2772-7.

[38] Hedman T, Kostuik J, Fernie G, et al. Design of an intervertebral disc prosthesis. Spine (Phila Pa 1976). 1991 ;16(6 Suppl):S256-60

[39] Idelberger K. Treatment of spinal tuberculosis Munch Med Wochenschr 1954;96(8):192-4.

[40] Charnley J. The classic: The bonding of prostheses to bone by cement. 1964. Clin Orthop Relat Res 2010;468(12):3149-59.

[41] Fathie K. Anterior cervical diskectomy and fusion with methylmethacrylate. Mt Sinai J Med 1994;61:246–247.

[42] Wilke HJ, Kettler A, Goetz C, et al. Subsidence resulting from simulated postoperative neck movements. Spine (Phila Pa 1976). 2000 Nov 1;25(21):2762-70.

[43] Kettler A, Wilke HJ, Claes L. Effect of neck movements on stability and subsidence in cervical interbody fusion, an in vitro study. J Neurosurg 2001 ;94(1 Suppl):97-107.

[44] Wilkinson JM, Eveleigh R, Hamer AJ, et al. Effect of mixing technique on the properties of acrylic bone-cement: a comparison of syringe and bowl mixing systems. J Arthroplasty 2000;15(5):663-7.

[45] Farrokhi MR, Torabinezhad S, Ghajar KA. Pilot study of a new acrylic cage in a dog cervical spine fusion model. J Spinal Disord Tech 2010;23(4):272-7.

[46] Kulkarni AG, Hee HT, Wong HK. Solis cage (PEEK) for anterior cervical fusion: preliminary radiological results with emphasis on fusion and subsidence. Spine J 2007;7(2):205-9.

Part 5

Oral and Maxillofacial Surgery

11

To Graft or Not to Graft? Evidence-Based Guide to Decision Making in Oral Bone Graft Surgery

Bernhard Pommer[1], Werner Zechner[1], Georg Watzek[1] and Richard Palmer[2]
[1]Department of Oral Surgery, Vienna Medical University
[2]Department of Restorative Dentistry, King's College London
[1]Austria
[2]UK

1. Introduction

Rehabilitation of the incomplete dentition by means of osseointegrated implants represents a highly predictable and widespread therapy. Advantages of oral implant treatment over conventional non-surgical prosthetic rehabilitation involve avoidance of removable dentures and tooth structure conservation of the remaining dentition. Implant placement necessitates sufficient bone quantity as well as bone quality, that may be compromised following tooth loss or trauma. Sufficient alveolar bone to host implants of 10 mm in length and 3-4 mm in diameter has been traditionally regarded as minimum requirements to allow bone-demanded implant placement. Three-dimensional bone morphology, however, may not permit favourable implant positioning. In the age of prosthetic-driven implant treatment, bone grafting procedures may be indicated not exclusively due to lack of bone volume, but to ensure favourable biomechanics and long-term esthetic outcome. A vast variety of treatment modalities have been suggested to increase alveolar bone volume and thus overcome the intrinsic limitations of oral implantology. Although success rates of various bone graft techniques are high, inherent disadvantages of augmentation procedures include prolonged treatment times, raised treatment costs and increased surgical invasion associated with patient morbidity and potential complications. Therefore, treatment tactics to obviate bone graft surgery are naturally preferred by both patients and surgeons. Non-grafting options, such as implants reduced in length and diameter or the use of computer-guided implant surgery, may on the other hand carry the risk of lower predictability and reduced long-term success. To graft or not to graft? – that is the question clinicians are facing day-to-day in oral implant rehabilitation.

Decision making in evidence-based implant dentistry involves diagnostic and therapeutic uncertainties, clinicians' heuristics and biases, patients' preferences and values, as well as cost considerations (Flemmig & Beikler, 2009). The evidence-based approach to oral healthcare emerged during the 1990s and was implemented in therapeutic decision making with the aim of maximizing the potential for successful patient care outcomes. The present book chapter offers an evaluation of implant treatment options in partially and completely edentulous patients to guide clinicians' decision making based on scientific evidence in contemporary literature. Therapeutic alternatives indicated for specific treatment situations are compiled and indications as well as limitations are outlined. Clinical investigations and systematic reviews comparing alternative bone graft techniques as well as trials comparing bone augmentation to non-grafting options are discussed. To allow for indirect comparison, studies using conventional implants (≥ 10 mm in length) as a reference standard (Griffin & Cheung, 2004) are also embraced. The highest level of evidence supporting therapeutic decisions is given using the Oxford 2011 Levels of Evidence classification system (Table 1). However, no down- or upgrading due to methodological study quality was performed, as the system was primarily used to indicate the presence (or absence) of (randomized) controlled trials on various treatment options.

LoE	Study design
1	Systematic review of randomized trials or n-of-1 trials
2	Randomized trial or observational study with dramatic effect
3	Non-randomized controlled cohort/follow-up study
4	Case-series, case-control studies, or historically controlled studies
5	Mechanism-based reasoning

Table 1. Level of evidence (LoE) classification system for treatment benefits according to the Oxford Centre for Evidence-Based Medicine (Howick et al., 2011)

Evidence on treatment options involving bone graft surgery was gained from recent systematic reviews and meta-analyses (Aghaloo & Moy, 2007; Att et al., 2009; Bernstein et al., 2006; Chao et al., 2010; Chiapasco et al., 2006, 2009; Donos et al., 2008; Emmerich et al., 2005; Esposito et al., 2009, 2010; Graziani et al., 2004; Jensen & Terheyden, 2009; Pjetursson et al. 2008; Rochietta et al., 2008; Stellingsma et al., 2004; Tan et al., 2008; Waasdorp & Reynolds, 2010) and supplemented by an electronic MEDLINE literature search (last search on 1st August 2011). Likewise, evidence on non-grafting treatment alternatives, i.e. short, tilted or zygomatic implants, was sought (Aparicio et al., 2008; Att et al., 2009; Del Fabbro et al., 2010; Esposito et al., 2005; Hagi et al., 2004; Jung et al., 2009; Kotosovilis et al., 2009; Pommer et al., 2011; Renouard & Nisand, 2006; Stellingsma et al., 2004).

2. Surgical techniques

This chapter addresses the six types of alveolar ridge augmentation: onlay block grafts, guided bone regeneration, sinus floor elevation, distraction osteogenesis, interpositional grafts and alveolar ridge expansion. As the present manuscript focuses on reconstruction of vertical or horizontal alveolar deficiencies, augmentation of post-extraction sockets (ridge preservation) and bone regeneration around immediate implants or implants presenting with bone defects following peri-implantitis are not included. Subsequently, surgical techniques to avoid oral bone graft surgery are covered: short implants, parasinusal tilted implants, zygomatic implants and alveolar nerve transposition.

2.1 Onlay block grafts

Onlay bone grafts are used for external augmentation of horizontal (veneer graft) or vertical alveolar ridge deficiencies, as well as combined defects (saddle graft). Compression screws are placed to fix bone blocks to the residual alveolar crest, that should be extensively perforated to increase blood supply to the host-graft interface (Lundgren et al., 2008). While autogenous bone is generally harvested from intra- or extraoral donor sites, the potential of allogeneic bone for onlay block grafts has also been documented (Waasdorp & Reynolds, 2010). Simultaneous implant placement can be an option only in vertical grafts, with the implants acting as osteosynthesis screws, and may carry the potential of shortening the healing phase (Chiapasco et al., 2006). The drawbacks, however, involve unpredictable graft resorption, higher risk of wound dehiscence and osseointegration failure, lower values of bone-to-implant contact and compromized implant position, thereby making the one-step procedure undesirable from a prosthetic point of view (Stellingsma et al., 2004). Implant survival and peri-implant bone levels have shown no significant differences following onlay block grafting compared to implants in native jawbone (LoE-4), however, these data include both horizontal and vertical grafts (Sbordone et al., 2009). A mean increase in horizontal and vertical dimension of 4.4 mm and 3.7 mm has been reported (Jensen & Terheyden, 2009) with rates of graft resorption of 10-50% (Chiapasco et al., 2009) and 29-42% (Bernstein et al., 2006), respectively (Figure 1a), dependent on the choice of bone harvest site. Complications involve wound dehiscence and total graft loss (Figure 1b) in 3.3% and 1.4%, respectively (Chiapasco et al., 2009). Controversy over the inclusion of barrier membranes to cover onlay grafts occurs from their potential negative effects in the event of wound dehiscence, as membrane exposure may result in passage of infectious agents along the membrane into the healing site (Bernstein et al., 2006). As true for all techniques of external bone augmentation, incidence of dehiscences is related to the ability to provide tension-free primary flap closure in cases of significant addition of graft volume.

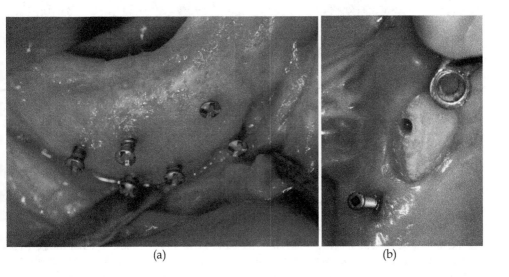

(a)   (b)

Fig. 1. Onlay block grafts: amount of graft resorption can be seen on fixation screws (a), graft loss following wound dehiscence (b) [pictures by Georg Watzek* and Thomas Bernhart*]

2.2 Guided bone regeneration

The concept of guided bone regeneration implies the use of cell-occlusive membranes for space provision over a vertical or horizontal defect, promoting the ingrowth of osteogenic cells while preventing migration of undesired cells from the overlying soft tissue (Block & Haggerty, 2009). Space maintenance by various particulate graft materials and the use of resorbable (Figure 2), non-resorbable as well as titanium-reinforced membranes has been described, while no indications regarding the choice of simultaneous vs. delayed implant placement have yet been defined (Chiapasco et al., 2006). No differences in implant survival rates following guided bone regeneration could be found (LoE-3) compared to implants in native jawbone, while observed significant differences in marginal bone resorption (1.4 mm vs. 1.2 mm) may not be of clinical relevance (Zitzmann et al., 2001). Mean increase in horizontal and vertical dimensions of 2.6 mm and 3.6 mm, respectively, has been reported (Jensen & Terheyden, 2009) with up to 40% of initial bone gain undergoing resorption thereafter (Chiapasco et al., 2009). Failures are mainly related to premature membrane exposure that has been seen in up to 38% of cases (Block & Haggerty, 2009) and may lead to infection and eventually partial or total loss of regenerated bone.

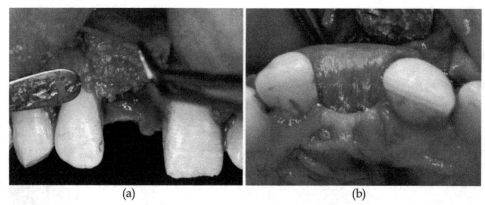

(a)   (b)

Fig. 2. Guided bone regeneration in the anterior maxilla using particulate graft material (a) and a resorbable membrane to increase horizontal ridge width (b) [pictures by Thomas Bernhart*]

2.3 Sinus floor elevation

Internal augmentation of the maxillary sinus to compensate for sinus pneumatization is based on the principle of guided bone regeneration using the sinus membrane as a natural barrier. Bone formation to allow osseointegration of delayed or simultaneously placed implants is initiated by coronal displacement of the maxillary sinus membrane with or without addition of bone (substitute) material. Membrane elevation is accomplished either via the lateral sinus wall (Figure 3), as described by Boyne in the 1960s, or via a transcrestal approach to the antrum, as decribed by Summers in the 1990s (Pjetursson et al., 2008). No significant difference in implant survival (LoE-3) could be found in sinus grafted bone vs. native jawbone (Graziani et al., 2004). The most frequent complication is the iatrogenic perforation of the sinus membrane in 10-20% of lateral approaches on average (Chiapasco et al., 2009; Pjetursson et al., 2008). Lateral sinus grafting can, however, be completed in a vast majority of cases by closing the perforation with resorbable materials. The main disadvantages of transcrestal elevation techniques are the uncertain diagnosis of membrane perforations and the lack of possibilities of repair (Pommer et al., 2009). Significantly greater bone graft heights (11.8 mm vs. 3.5 mm, 79 patients, LoE-3) have been obtained using the lateral vs. transcrestal approach (Zitzmann & Schärer, 1998), yet recent modifications to the osteotome-technique, such as membrane elevation by inflation of a balloon catheter and the use of hydraulic or gel pressure, have shown the potential to accomplish greater elevation heights despite the minimally invasive approach (Pommer & Watzek, 2009). Postoperative sinusitis may occur at a mean rate of 3% and 1% following lateral and transcrestal augmentation, respectively (Pjetursson et al., 2008; Tan et al., 2008). Spread of infection to intracranial structures via the cavernous sinus is a rare yet serious complication. Total graft loss has been recorded at a mean rate of 2% in lateral sinus floor augmentation (Pjetursson et al. 2008).

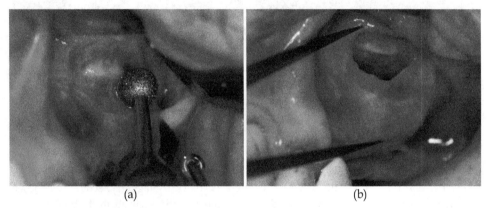

(a)   (b)

Fig. 3. Sinus floor augmentation via a lateral approach (a) to gain sufficient bone height (b) for implant placement in the posterior maxilla [pictures by Werner Zechner*]

2.4 Distraction osteogenesis

Distraction osteogenesis relies on the biologic phenomenon that new bone fills in the gap defect created when two bone segments are slowly separated under tension. One week after osteotomy and distractor placement (latency period) distraction of segments is advanced at a rate of 0.5-1 mm per day until the desired separation is reached (Figure 4). A consolidation period of 5 days per mm space created should be respected before device removal and implant placement (Bernstein et al., 2006). Despite inherent disadvantages (need for daily activation, compromised speech, eating and appearance) the procedure offers unique possibilities: vertical bone gain of 3-20 mm may be accomplished without the use of graft material and additional mucosal grafting is obviated as the soft tissue follows bone distraction (Chiapasco et al., 2006). However, complications include partial relapse of initial bone height (8%), change of distraction vector (8%), basal bone or segment fracture (3%), fracture of distraction device (2%), incomplete distraction (2%), transient paresthesia (2%) and total failure in 1% of cases on average (Chiapasco et al., 2009). Distraction osteogenesis does generally not allow correction of narrow ridges, which may only be possible by overdistraction of the segment and secondary height reduction until adequate bone width is obtained. Overcorrection may, however, give rise to surrounding tissue tears or ischemia (Bernstein et al., 2006).

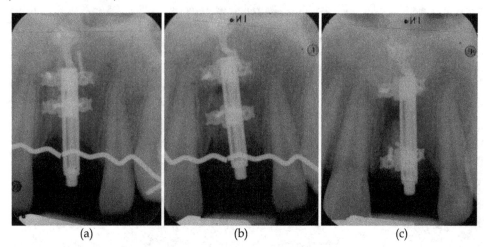

(a)   (b)   (c)

Fig. 4. Distraction osteogenesis in the anterior maxilla: (a) latency phase after distractor placement, (b) distraction phase, (c) consolidation phase after desired separation is reached [pictures by Georg Watzek* and Thomas Bernhart*]

2.5 Interpositional grafts

Just as distraction osteogenesis, interpositional bone grafts (also known as sandwich grafts) are exclusively used for treatment of vertical defects (Block & Haggerty, 2009). By contrast, the osteotomized bone segment is not distracted but initially secured in its final position using osteosynthesis plates. Surgical techniques in the mandible (frequently using bone substitute materials to augment the gap) show large differences to those in the edentulous maxilla, where interpositional autologous grafts are placed after Le Fort I osteotomy and maxillary down-fracture (Chiapasco et al., 2006). Wound dehiscences in 4% of mandibular grafts compare to overall complication rates of up to 10% following Le Fort I osteotomies in the maxilla including postoperative sinusitis (3%), wound dehiscence (3%), partial graft loss (3%), midpalatal fracture (2%) and total graft failure in 1% on average (Chiapasco et al., 2009). Rare complications involve massive hemorrhage and blindness. Due to unpredictable bone resorption and plate removal at implant placement, one-stage procedures are generally not preferred in both maxillary and mandibular interpositional grafting (Att et al., 2009).

2.6 Alveolar ridge expansion

Alveolar ridge expansion (also known as bone splitting technique) represents the horizontal equivalent to vertical distraction or interpositional grafting. Following crestal osteotomy the buccal cortex is gently expanded against the lingual plate using osteotomes of increasing diameters to allow implants to be placed in between (Figure 5). The residual gap created may be filled with graft material but seems to undergo spontaneous ossification (Chiapasco et al., 2006). Bone splitting of knife-edge ridges is only possible if the buccal and lingual cortices are separated by spongy bone. Gain in horizontal bone width has been found to average 4 mm (Holzclaw et al., 2010) while malfracture of the buccal plate has been reported in 4-22% of cases (Sohn et al., 2004; Jensen et al., 2009). Due to the lower bone density and thinner cortical plates success rates may certainly be higher in the maxilla. No significant differences (LoE-4) in implant survival and peri-implant bone levels have been observed following alveolar ridge expansion compared to conventional implant placement (Danza et al., 2009), however, there is a paucity of data with regard to the stability of initial bone volume as well as marginal bone resorption in reaction to the surgical trauma of expansion.

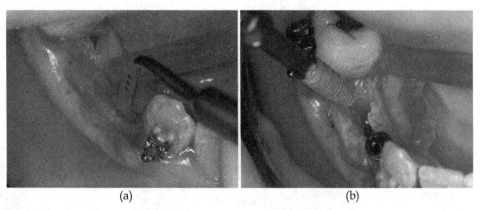

(a)   (b)

Fig. 5. Alveolar ridge expansion in the posterior mandible: (a) crestal osteotomy using piezoelectric saw, (b) implant placement following ridge splitting [pictures by Dieter Busenlechner*]

2.7 Short implants

It has been an axiom in implant dentistry that longer implants guarantee lower failure rates, although a linear relationship between implant length and success has never been proven. While conventional dental implants of at least 10 mm in length are considered the reference standard of implant therapy (Griffin & Cheung, 2004) positive clinical results with shorter implants have increased the interest in this promising technique to avoid invasive bone graft surgery. Strategies to increase the surface area of short implants include the use of rough-surfaced implants and wider implant diameters, however, literature results support the hypothesis that implant diameter increase can not compensate for length reduction (Maló et al., 2007; Pommer et al., 2011). Short implants may be splinted to each other and/or longer implants in fixed partial dentures to enhance force distribution. A tendency of short implant failures to occur within the first year of prosthetic loading has been observed (das Neves et al., 2006) and long-term effects of peri-implant bone resorption may also differ significantly and require investigation. Meta-analyses of observational studies (LoE-3) did not reveal differences between short (7-9 mm) and conventional (≥ 10 mm) rough-surfaced implants regarding their survival (Kotsovilis et al., 2009) as well as one-year success rates (Pommer et al., 2011).

2.8 Parasinusal tilted implants

One way to avoid short implants as well as bone graft surgery is the use of tilted implants, i.e. implants with an inclination greater than 15° (up to 35°) towards the occlusal plane (Friberg, 2008). No difference (LoE-3) in early failure rates and marginal bone resorption could be found between tilted and axial implants (Del Fabbro et al., 2010). Implants in the anterior maxilla as well as pterygoid implants in the maxillary tuberosity may both be tilted (Figure 6a) to avoid the sinus cavity and allow for greater implant lengths without bone augmentation. Parasinusal tilting may further reduce the length of cantilever segments thus improving biomechanic load distribution (Block & Haggerty, 2009). With guided implant surgery, the placement of tilted implants has become not only easier and less invasive from a surgical point of view (Att et al., 2009) but also more efficient and predictable from the prosthetic viewpoint (Figure 6b). The introduction of computed tomography, implant planning software and CAD/CAM technology have undoubtedly been important achievements to provide optimal 3D implant positioning with respect to both prosthetic and anatomical parameters (Jung et al., 2009).

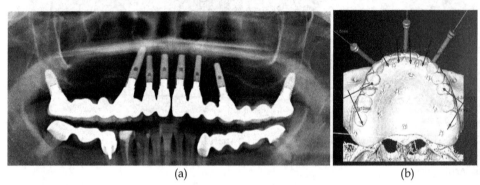

(a)   (b)

Fig. 6. Parasinusal placement of tilted implants in the atrophic maxilla (a) using CT-based implant treatment planning software (b) [pictures by Werner Zechner*]

2.9 Zygomatic implants

Zygomatic implants have mainly been used in the rehabilitation of severely resorbed or partially resected maxillae in combination with premaxillary implants as an alternative to bone grafting (Friberg, 2008). Complications involve postoperative sinusitis in up to 14% of cases as well as temporary paresthesia, epistaxis, facial and periorbital hematoma and orbital penetration (Block & Haggerty, 2009). While palatal emergence (up to 12 mm medial to the ridge) is frequent with zygomatic implants and may cause prosthetic difficulties (Att et al., 2009), their generally posterior position has been shown to cause problems with oral hygiene. Peri-implant bleeding, soft tissue hyperplasia and increased pocket depths have been recorded in up to 45% of cases (Aparicio et al., 2008) and may result in oroantral fistula formation and subsequent maxillary sinusitis (Figure 7). Recent developments such as extrasinusal placement and the use of CT-based surgical stents may help to overcome these problems, however, it should be considered that mean angular deviations of 4° using mucosa-supported templates (Jung et al., 2009; Vasak et al., 2011) may result in significantly higher imprecision at the apex of 30 to 55 mm long implants.

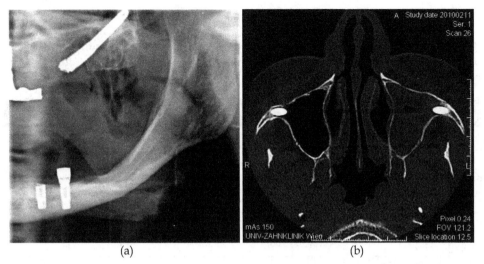

Fig. 7. Marginal bone loss around zygomatic implants (a) may lead to oroantral fistula formation and subsequent maxillary sinusitis (b) [pictures by Georg Watzek*]

2.10 Alveolar nerve transposition

Transposition of the inferior alveolar nerve consists of exposing the neurovascular bundle from a lateral approach with its release from the mandibular canal, and repositioning it laterally, allowing implants to be placed as far as the inferior border of the mandible (Block & Haggerty, 2009). Drawbacks of this procedure include a high incidence of neurosensory disturbances of up to 90%, risk of mandibular fracture and increased crown lengths associated with compromised implant esthetics (Chrcanovic & Custódio, 2009).

2.11 Comparison of surgical techniques

Table 2 provides an overview of implant survival, augmentation success and complication rates of bone graft techniques and non-grafting options reported in contemporary literature. On the basis of between-study comparison, however, it is difficult to demonstrate that one particular surgical procedure offers superior outcomes (Chiapasco et al., 2006). It remains doubtful whether any strong evidence to support treatment decisions may be produced by non-comparative follow-up investigations, that oral implant research has focused on during the last decades.

Post-extraction alveolar ridge resorption follows a predictable pattern (Cawood & Howell, 1988) changing its shape from high-well-rounded (generally not requiring bone grafts), to knife-edged (corrected by horizontal augmentation) and low-well-rounded ridges (calling for vertical grafts). It is essential to consider the initial clinical situation in this comparison, as horizontal bone grafts have been shown to be more predictable (Bernstein et al., 2006) and no surgical technique suits any given defect. Significantly greater horizontal bone gain has been reported using onlay block grafts (4.0 mm vs. 2.7 mm, 30 patients, LoE-3) vs. guided bone regeneration (Chiapasco et al., 1999). Augmentation of vertical bone height using distraction osteogenesis has been demonstrated to yield significantly lower graft resorption prior to implant placement (0.3 mm vs. 0.6 mm, 17 patients, LoE-2) vs. onlay grafts (Chiapasco et al., 2007) as well as significantly higher implant success and lower marginal bone resorption (93% vs. 64%, 1.4 mm vs. 1.9 mm, 21 patients, LoE-2) vs. guided bone regeneration (Chiapasco et al., 2004).

Treatment option	Mean implant survival rate	Mean gain in height/width	Mean graft resorption	Mean rate of complications
Onlay block graft	89% (60-100)			
horizontal	99% (97-100)	5 mm	22%	4%
vertical	85% (76-100)	4 mm	38%	30%
Guided bone regeneration	96% (77-100)			
horizontal	98% (77-100)	3 mm	14%	40%
vertical	98% (92-100)	4 mm	n.d.	21%
Lateral sinus floor elevation	95% (60-100)	12 mm	17%	25%
Transcrestal sinus floor elevation	96% (83-100)	4 mm	18%	5%
Distraction osteogenesis	96% (88-100)	7 mm	11%	25%
Le Fort I + interpositional graft	88% (60-95)	n.d.	n.d.	12%
Mandibular interpositional graft	92% (90-95)	6 mm	13%	4%
Alveolar ridge expansion	94% (91-97)	4 mm	14%	19%
Short implants	97% (74-100)	no graft	no graft	no complications
Parasinusal tilted implants	98% (89-100)	no graft	no graft	no complications
Zygomatic implants	98% (82-100)	no graft	no graft	14%
Alveolar nerve transposition	93% (88-100)	no graft	no graft	23%

Table 2. Results of systematic reviews reporting on treatment outcomes of various bone graft techniques and non-grafting options (n.d. = no data).

It does, however, seem problematic to compare implant success following different surgical techniques if both maxillary and mandibular sites are included. As conventional implants (≥ 10 mm) in native jawbone show diverging failure rates in the anterior maxilla (2.1% [$CI^{95\%}$ 1.7-2.7], n=3607), posterior maxilla (2.5% [$CI^{95\%}$ 2.0-3.0], n=4039), anterior mandible (1.1% [$CI^{95\%}$ 0.9-1.4], n=5797) and posterior mandible (1.7% [$CI^{95\%}$ 1.4-2.1], n=5640) even after 1 year of prosthetic loading (Pommer et al., 2011), it should be considered that regional differences may very well exist in grafted bone. Selection of the appropriate surgical technique should not only be based on the location in the mouth (Aghaloo & Moy, 2007) but also on complete vs. partial edentulous patient situations. The next two chapters discuss evidence on treatment decisions in complete and partial edentulism. Treatment alternatives based on the shortened arch concept, cantilever or implant/tooth-supported bridges and subperiosteal or transosteal implants are not embraced. Trials comparing different bone (substitute) materials, types of barrier membranes or fixation screws, simultaneous vs. delayed implant placement, implant macro- and microstructure, loading protocols or types of prosthetic restorations as well as uncontrolled studies are given insufficient attention.

3. Bone grafting in complete edentulism

The main goal of implant treatment in edentulous patients is to provide either fixed full-arch bridges or retention and stability to their removable dentures. Both approaches may require bone graft surgery, however, various factors such as patient age and health, surgical hazard and opposing dentition should be considered. Implant-supported rehabilitation may, on the other hand, prevent further alveolar ridge resorption and not only improve oral health and patient satisfaction, but also patients' nutritional status and quality of life in general. Nongrafting options may generally be preferred in cases of previous graft failure, general medical contraindications to bone graft surgery or to avoid maxillary sinus floor elevation in patients with prominent sinus septa or a history of chronic sinusitis.

3.1 Treatment options in the edentulous maxilla

In the severely atrophic edentulous maxilla, centripetal alveolar resorption, the presence of maxillary sinuses, nasal fossa and incisive foramen, along with low bone quality, complicate implant treatment. Insufficient bone height may be related to vertical resorption of the alveolar ridge, sinus pneumatization, or a combination of both. In cases of severe increase in interarch distance, external rather than internal bone augmentation may be indicated to avoid compromised crown-to-implant ratios as well as unfavourable deviation of implant positions towards the palate (Chiapasco et al., 2006). Treatment options in the edentulous maxilla involve onlay block grafts, guided bone regeneration, lateral sinus floor elevation, interpositional grafts in combination with Le Fort I osteotomy, parasinusal tilting and zygomatic implants (Table 3), however, a combination of graft techniques may at times be necessary to optimize implant placement from a functional and esthetic point of view (Chiapasco et al., 2006). Lateral cephalograms should be taken with the removable dentures in place in order to determine jaw relationship and estimate proper lip support (Lundgren et al., 2008). Le Fort I osteotomy may be indicated in patients with a markedly reverse jaw relationship and severe vertical deficiency, while onlay grafts may be preferred if an inverted jaw relationship is combined with a knife-edge ridge (Att et al., 2009). Grafting of the nasal floor combined with onlay blocks may be indicated in case of short vertical height of the anterior maxilla (Lundgren et al., 2008). Due to relevant patient morbidity interpositional grafts should be limited to severe cases, in which other techniques are not able to re-establish an acceptable intermaxillary relationship (Att et al., 2009). No significant difference (LoE-3) regarding implant survival could be seen following onlay block grafts vs. lateral sinus floor elevation (Wiltfang et al., 2005) as well as vs. interpositional grafts in conjunction with Le Fort I osteotomy (Lundgren et al., 2008). No significant differences (LoE-3) in bone-to-implant contacts and newly formed bone around microimplants retrieved 6-14 months after onlay vs. interpositional grafting were observed (Sjöström et al., 2006). To date, no information is available on the outcome of short implants or transcrestal sinus floor elevation in the edentulous maxilla (Att et al., 2009). No controlled studies on guided bone regeneration, zygomatic implants and parasinusal tilted implants could be identified.

3.2 Treatment options in the edentulous mandible

The atrophic edentulous mandible, by contrast, may predominantly present conditions that are compatible with implant placement. Avoidance of bone augmentation has even been suggested as long as the intraforaminal region is more than 5 mm in height and at least 6 mm in width (Keller, 1995). Bone augmentation should be limited to severely atrophic cases with the risk of fatigue mandibular fracture (Chiapasco et al., 2009). Treatment options for vertical heights <10 mm involve onlay block grafts (Figure 8), guided bone regeneration, distraction osteogenesis, interpositional grafts as well as short implants (Table 4). No significant difference (LoE-3) in early implant failure (OR 0.7 [CI$^{95\%}$ 0.2-2.4]) could be found between short (7-9 mm) and conventional (≥ 10 mm) rough-surfaced implants (Pommer et al., 2011). Significantly lower implant success (LoE-3) and more negative experience of the surgical phase was seen in interpositional grafts of the interforaminal region vs. short implants (Stellingsma et al., 2003), yet 30% of these implants were 11 mm in length and may thus not be regarded as short. No controlled studies on any other bone graft techniques could be identified.

Bone graft treatment options	Indications & Limitations	LoE
Onlay block graft	No inherent limitations	3
Guided bone regeneration	No inherent limitations	4
Lateral sinus floor elevation	No inherent limitations	3
Le Fort I + interpositional graft	Limited to severe atrophy or intermaxillary discrepancy	3
Nongrafting treatment options	Indications & Limitations	LoE
Parasinusal tilted implants	Limited by residual bone volume in premaxillary and retromolar regions	4
Zygomatic implants	Placed in conjunction with premaxillary implants	4

Table 3. Treatment options in the edentulous maxilla

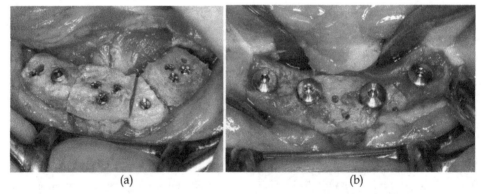

(a)   (b)

Fig. 8. Onlay bone grafting of the edentulous mandible (a) to facilitate interforaminal implant placement (b) [pictures by Markus Hof* and Gabriella Eisenmenger*]

Bone graft treatment options	Indications & Limitations	LoE
Onlay block graft	No inherent limitations	4
Guided bone regeneration	No inherent limitations	4
Distraction osteogenesis	Limited to a minimum residual bone height of 6 mm in the presence of residual alveolar width of at least 4 mm	4
Interpositional graft	Limited to a minimum residual bone height of 6 mm in the presence of residual alveolar width of at least 4 mm	3
Nongrafting treatment options	Indications & Limitations	LoE
Short implants	Indicated in cases of at least 5-7 mm bone height	3

Table 4. Treatment options in the edentulous mandible

4. Bone grafting in partial edentulism

In contrast to completely edentulous jaws, partial edentulism presents with a vast variety of dentition patterns including single-tooth and intermediate gaps as well as posterior free-end situations. Treatment decisions are therefore more complex and non-surgical alternatives may involve non-removable restorations such as fixed partial dentures, cantilever and resin-bonded bridges. Just by their presence, residual teeth may sometimes complicate treatment planning in cases of partial edentulism (Friberg, 2008). Depending on their periodontal and general condition, exceptional extraction of the residual dentition and thus transformation of partial into complete edentulism may at times prove advantageous in terms of avoiding bone graft surgery or even lowering treatment costs.

4.1 Deficient anterior maxillary sites

Bone resorption in the anterior maxilla following tooth loss occurs early (50% during the first 12 months) but mainly in the horizontal direction with most of the bone loss on the buccal aspect (Att et al., 2009). Treatment options for horizontal deficiencies involve onlay block grafts, guided bone regeneration and alveolar ridge expansion (Table 5). No significant differences (LoE-2) regarding implant survival, marginal gingiva and bone levels as well as implant esthetics (Meijndert et al., 2007) could be found between onlay block grafts vs. guided bone regeneration. Bone biopsies at implant placement revealed no differences in total bone volume and marrow connective tissue volume (Meijndert et al., 2005). No controlled study on alveolar ridge expansion in anterior maxillary sites could be identified.

Bone graft treatment options	Indications & Limitations	LoE
Onlay block graft	No inherent limitations	2
Guided bone regeneration	No inherent limitations	2
Alveolar ridge expansion	Limited to a minimum residual bone width of 4 mm	4

Table 5. Treatment options for horizontal deficiency of the anterior maxilla

In less frequent cases requiring vertical bone augmentation onlay block grafts, guided bone regeneration and distraction osteogenesis may be considered. Additional soft tissue grafts may be obviated by the use of distraction osteogenesis (Figure 9), however, ridge defects of only 1 or 2 teeth in width have been associated with higher complication rates (Jensen et al., 2002). No controlled studies on any treatment option could be identified. Short implants do not seem to represent a good option in the anterior maxilla, as increased crown lengths lead to significantly compromised implants esthetics (Chiapasco et al., 2009). Enlarged incisive foramina may at times require grafting prior to implant placement in central maxillary incisor positions (Ragheobar et al., 2010).

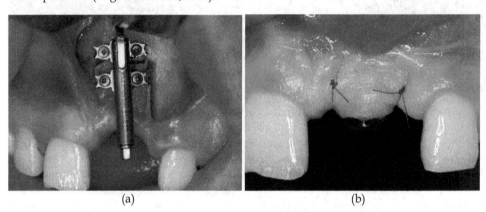

(a)   (b)

Fig. 9. Distraction osteogenesis in the vertically deficient anterior maxilla (a) to avoid additional soft tissue grafting (b) [pictures by Georg Watzek* and Thomas Bernhart*]

4.2 Deficient posterior maxillary sites

While horizontal defects are predominant in the anterior maxilla, the partial edentulous posterior maxilla presents with sufficient subantral bone width of 6 mm on average (Att et al., 2009) but residual alveolar ridge heights of less than 5 mm in 43% of cases (Lundgren et al., 1996). While short implants may not be an option in these cases, there is no evidence to recommend a minimum bone height that would contraindicate lateral or transcrestal sinus floor elevation (Chiapasco et al., 2009). Meta-regression revealed a significant trend of less implant failures in greater bone heights following lateral sinus floor elevation (Chao et al., 2010). No effect could be seen in transcrestal techniques (due to the lack of data below 4 mm), however, a minimum height of 4-6 mm is generally suggested (Tan et al., 2008). It is difficult to evaluate whether the support is offered by the graft or the native jawbone, when comparing survival rates in sinus grafted bone to those of short implants (Chiapasco et al., 2006). No significant difference (LoE-3) in early implant failure (OR 0.9 [CI[95%] 0.7-4.2]) could be found between short (7-9 mm) and conventional (≥ 10 mm) rough-surfaced implants (Pommer et al., 2011), however, compromised crown-to-implant ratios may give rise to long-term biomechanical overload (Block & Haggerty, 2009). Conventional implants did neither show significant differences regarding implant survival (LoE-3) when compared to transcrestal sinus floor elevation, yet only 28% of simultaneous implants were placed in residual bone heights of 7-9 mm (Gabbert et al., 2009) and therefore indirect comparison was not anticipated.

Conventional implants placed following lateral sinus floor elevation (Figure 10) did not show higher survival rates (LoE-2) vs. 5 mm short implants (Esposito et al., 2011) as well as vs. 8 mm short implants placed in conjunction with transcrestal sinus floor elevation (Cannizzaro et al., 2009). No controlled studies on parasinusal tilted or zygomatic implants in the partially edentulous posterior maxilla could be found (Friberg, 2008). The application of distraction osteogenesis in the posterior maxilla is limited by the proximity of the maxillary sinus (Bernstein et al., 2006). No controlled studies on external augmentation using onlay block grafts or guided bone regeneration in the partially edentulous posterior maxilla to correct for increased interarch distance could be identified (Table 6).

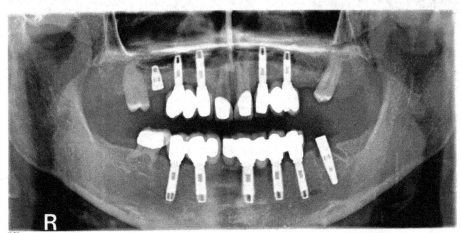

Fig. 10. Oligodontia patient showing two treatment modalities for deficient posterior maxillary sites: short implant (8 mm) without bone graft (right side) vs. sinus floor augmentation prior to the placement of longer implants (left side) [picture by Bernhard Pommer*]

Bone graft treatment options	Indications & Limitations	LoE
Onlay block graft	No inherent limitations	4
Guided bone regeneration	No inherent limitations	4
Lateral sinus floor elevation	No inherent limitations	2
Transcrestal sinus floor elevation	Residual bone height of 4-6 mm suggested	2
Nongrafting treatment options	Indications & Limitations	LoE
Short implants	Indicated in cases of at 5-7 mm bone height	2
Parasinusal tilted implants	Limited by residual bone volume in premaxillary and retromolar regions	4
Zygomatic implants	Placed in conjunction with premaxillary implants	4

Table 6. Treatment options for vertical deficiency of the posterior maxilla

4.3 Deficient anterior mandibular sites

Similar to the anterior maxilla, edentulous anterior mandibular ridges are often knife-edged in shape. Treatment options for horizontal deficiencies involve onlay block grafts, guided bone regeneration and alveolar ridge expansion (Table 7). Reduction of ridge height until adequate bone width is obtained and subsequent apical implant placement may be a non-grafting option but is associated with increased crown length and compromised implant esthetics. Compared to the anterior maxilla, however, more patients may accept an esthetic compromise. No controlled studies on any treatment option could be identified.

Bone graft treatment options	Indications & Limitations	LoE
Onlay block graft	No inherent limitations	4
Guided bone regeneration	No inherent limitations	4
Alveolar ridge expansion	Limited to a minimum residual bone width of 4 mm	4
Non-grafting treatment options	Indications & Limitations	LoE
Apical implant placement	Limited indications due to compromised implant esthetics	4

Table 7. Treatment options for horizontal deficiency of the anterior mandible

In less frequent cases requiring vertical bone augmentation onlay block grafts, guided bone regeneration, distraction osteogenesis as well as (esthetically compromised) apical implant placement may be considered. No controlled studies on any treatment option could be identified.

4.4 Deficient posterior mandibular sites

The obvious limitation of implant placement in the posterior mandible is the presence of the inferior alveolar nerve (Block & Haggerty, 2009). Due to denture-related alveolar resorption, predominantly low-well-rounded ridge shapes can be found. Treatment options for vertical deficiencies involve onlay block grafts, guided bone regeneration, distraction osteogenesis, interpositional grafts, short implants and transposition of the inferior alveolar nerve (Table 8). No significant difference (LoE-3) in early implant failure (OR 0.5 [CI$^{95\%}$ 0.1-2.3]) could be found between short (7-9 mm) and conventional ($\geq$ 10 mm) rough-surfaced implants (Pommer et al., 2011), however, unfavourable crown-to-implant ratios may not only compromise implant esthetics but also give rise to long-term biomechanical overload (Figure 11) depending on interarch distance (Block & Haggerty, 2009). No significant

Bone graft treatment options	Indications & Limitations	LoE
Onlay block graft	No inherent limitations	2
Guided bone regeneration	No inherent limitations	4
Distraction osteogenesis	Limited to a minimum residual bone height of 6 mm	2
Interpositional graft	Limited to a minimum residual bone height of 6 mm	2
Nongrafting treatment options	Indications & Limitations	LoE
Short implants	Indicated in cases of at 5-7 mm bone height	2
Alveolar nerve transposition	Limited indications due to risk of nerve damage	4

Table 8. Treatment options for vertical deficiency of the posterior mandible

differences (LoE-2) regarding implant survival were found comparing interpositional grafts vs. 7 mm short implants (Felice et al., 2010), vs. 5 mm short implants (Esposito et al., 2011), vs. distraction osteogenesis (Bianchi et al., 2008) or vs. onlay block grafts (Felice et al., 2009). However, interpositional grafts showed significantly less gain in bone height (5.8 mm vs. 10 mm, 12 patients) vs. distraction osteogenesis (Bianchi et al., 2008), but significantly less bone resorption (0.5 mm vs. 2.8 mm, 20 patients) vs. onlay block grafts (Felice et al., 2009). No controlled studies on guided bone regeneration and inferior alveolar nerve transposition could be identified.

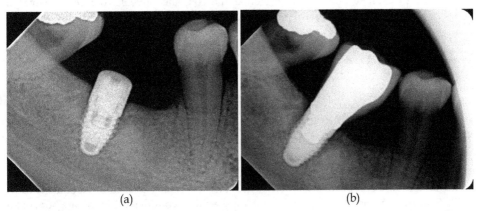

(a)   (b)

Fig. 11. Short implants (8 mm) in the posterior mandible (a) may result in compromised crown-to-implant ratios and long-term biomechanical overload (b) as well as esthetic compromise [pictures by Bernhard Pommer*]

In less frequent cases requiring horizontal bone augmentation onlay block grafts, guided bone regeneration, alveolar ridge expansion as well as ridge height reduction prior to apical placement of short implants may be considered. No significant differences (LoE-3) regarding implant success, peri-implant bone loss and implant stability could be found between buccal onlay bone grafts vs. conventional implant placement (Özkan et al., 2007). No controlled studies on any treatment option could be identified.

3. Conclusion and future research implications

Although several bone graft techniques as well as nongrafting treatment options can be considered well documented for different indications (Jensen & Terheyden, 2009), there is significant lack of comparative effectiveness research (CER) to guide decision making in oral bone graft surgery. While some surgical options have been compared in randomized (LoE-2) or non-randomized controlled trials (LoE-3), evidence on other treatment alternatives is based on between-study comparison. Even indirect comparison of study results could not provide further evidence. No long-term investigation comparing all available treatment options for any completely or partially edentulous situation could be identified. Priority may be given to procedures that appear less invasive and carry a lower risk of complications (Esposito et al., 2009).

Alveolar ridge deficiencies have traditionally been classified as horizontal (class I), vertical (class II) or combined (class III) defects (Seibert, 1983). Since the choice of surgical approach as well as the sequence of bone healing is largely dependent on the extent of the defect (Att et al., 2009), parameters concerning the initial clinical situation should be presented in more detail. Residual bone height is routinely investigated as an influencing variable in sinus floor augmentation trials, yet may not only affect treatment outcomes but also the choice of surgical technique. Recently, a modified classification (distinguishing 9 categories) has been presented to describe the atrophy-related initial situation of the edentulous maxilla and its impact on treatment decisions illustrated (Chiapasco et al., 2008).

In comparing treatment options for horizontal and combined alveolar defects, however, it seems relevant to evaluate initial bone morphology in 2 or even 3 dimensions. Not only residual bone but also graft extent should be described in terms of volume (Chiapasco et al., 2006) to allow more accurate evaluation of treatment success and recommendation of well-defined surgical protocols according to the initial situation (Chiapasco et al., 2008). Other confounding variables to be accounted for may be patient- (age, gender, smoking, comorbidity), implant- (dimension, micro-/macrostructure, implant bed preparation technique, loading protocol) or prosthetic- (type and fixation, crown-to-implant ratio, occlusal table) or outcome-related (success criteria, radiographic imaging, implant- vs. patient-based analysis).

Meaningful comparison of treatment outcomes should include implant success, long-term marginal bone resorption as well as graft success. However, only 9% of studies on oral bone augmentation measure the amount of bone gain and its stability over time (Aghaloo & Moy, 2007). Three-dimensional radiographic imaging should be considered to evaluate horizontal grafts. Peri-implant mucosal health and pocket depths may be crucial to long-term success. However, it should be kept in mind that all these clinical and radiological measures just represent surrogate endpoints for patient-related outcomes, i.e. long-term function and esthetics. Implant esthetics are considered essential in the anterior maxilla, while their impact on treatment decisions in other jaw regions remains unclear. However, no consensus on evaluation methodology has been reached yet and esthetic indices used have shown poor correlation to subjective patients' opinion (Meijndert et al., 2007). Patient-based outcome assessment may involve overall satisfaction with treatment results (most commonly rated on visual analogue scale), patients' perception of the surgical intervention and its impact on oral health-related quality of life (OHRQoL). The Oral Health Impact Profile (OHIP) has been established as a validated instrument (Slade & Spencer, 1994), however, most studies do not evaluate OHRQoL or do not draw within-subject comparison between pre- and post-treatment conditions. Cost-efficiency analyses, in particular, may benefit substantially from OHRQoL data. Finally, outcome assessment should embrace rates of surgical as well as prosthetic complications. As characteristics of possible complications vary significantly between surgical techniques, as described in chapter 2, comparison is inherently difficult (Esposito et al., 2005) and further complicates treatment choice.

The GRADE (Grading of Recommendations, Assessment, Development and Evaluation) Working Group has focused on addressing methodological shortcomings in evidence-based health care and developing a common, sensible approach (Guyatt et al., 2011). International organisations such as the Cochrane Collaboration and World Health Organisation have provided input into the development and started using it. Treatment recommendations are based on an overall level of scientific evidence, that has been defined as the lowest evidence of all treatment outcomes that seem crucial. Outcomes are considered crucial if they are likely to influence treatment decisions. To date no definition of crucial outcomes of implant rehabilitation has been attempted. The concept of evidence-based decision making in oral bone graft surgery seems to provide future research implications without measure.

4. Acknowledgment

We gratefully acknowledge the contributions of Professor Marco Esposito (Cochrane Oral Health Group, University of Manchester, UK), Professor Gordan H. Guyatt (GRADE Working Group, McMaster University, ON, Canada), Professor Jeremy Howick (Oxford Centre for Evidence-Based Medicine, UK), Professor Mike T. John (University of Minnesota, MN, United States), Professor Tim Newton (King's College London, UK) and Professor Michael A. Pogrel (University of California, San Francisco, CA, United States).

5. References

Aghaloo, T.L. & Moy, P.K. (2007) Which hard tissue augmentation techniques are the most successful in furnishing bony support for implant placement?. *The International Journal of Oral & Maxillofacial Implants*, Vol.22, Suppl, (December 2007), pp. 49-70, ISSN 0882-2786

Aparicio, C., Ouazzani, W. & Hatano, N. (2008) The use of zygomatic implants for prosthetic rehabilitation of the severely resorbed maxilla. *Periodontology 2000*, Vol.47, No.1, (June 2008), pp. 162-171, ISSN 0906-6713

Att, W., Bernhart, J. & Strub, J.R. (2009) Fixed rehabilitation of the edentulous maxilla: possibilities and clinical outcome. *Journal of Oral and Maxillofacial Surgery*, Vol.67, No.11 (Suppl), (November 2009), pp. 60-73, ISSN 0278-2391

Bernstein, S., Cooke, J., Fotek, P. & Wang, H.L. (2006) Vertical bone augmentation: where are we now? *Implant Dentistry*, Vol.15, No.3, (September 2006), pp. 219-228, ISSN 1056-6163

Bianchi, A., Felice, P., Lizio, G. & Marchetti, C. (2008) Alveolar distraction osteogenesis versus inlay bone grafting in posterior mandibular atrophy: a prospective study. *Oral Surgery, Oral Medicine, Oral Pathology, Oral Radiology, and Endodontics*, Vol.105, No.3, (March 2008), pp. 282-292, ISSN 1079-2104

Block, M.S. & Haggerty, C.J. (2009) Interpositional osteotomy for posterior mandible ridge augmentation. *Journal of Oral and Maxillofacial Surgery*, Vol.67, Suppl, (November 2009), pp. 31-39, ISSN 0278-2391

Cannizzaro, G., Felice, P., Leone, M., Viola, P. & Esposito, M. (2009) Early loading of implants in the atrophic posterior maxilla: lateral sinus lift with autogenous bone and Bio-Oss versus crestal mini sinus lift and 8-mm hydroxyapatite-coated implants. A randomised controlled clinical trial. *European Journal of Oral Implantology*, Vol.2, No.1, (Spring 2009), pp. 25-38, ISSN 1756-2406

Cawood, J.I. & Howell, R.A. (1988) A classification of the edentulous jaws. *International Journal of Oral and Maxillofacial Surgery*, Vol.17, No.4, (August 1988), pp. 232-236, ISSN 0901-5027

Chao, Y.L., Chen, H.H., Mei, C.C., Tu, Y.K. & Lu, H.K. (2010) Meta-regression analysis of the initial bone height for predicting implant survival rates of two sinus elevation procedures. *Journal of Clinical Periodontology*, Vol.37, No.5, (May 2008), pp. 456-465, ISSN 0303-6979

Chiapasco, M., Abati, S., Romeo, E. & Vogel, G. (1999) Clinical outcome of autogenous bone blocks or guided bone regeneration with e-PTFE membranes for the reconstruction of narrow edentulous ridges. *Clinical Oral Implants Research*, Vol.10, No.4, (August 1999), pp. 278-288, ISSN 0905-7161

Chiapasco, M., Romeo, E., Casentini, P. & Rimondini, L. (2004) Alveolar distraction osteogenesis vs. vertical guided bone regeneration for the correction of vertically deficient edentulous ridges: a 1-3-year prospective study on humans. *Clinical Oral Implants Research*, Vol.15, No.1, (February 2004), pp. 82-95, ISSN 0905-7161

Chiapasco, M., Zaniboni, M. & Boisco, M. (2006) Augmentation procedures for the rehabilitation of deficient edentulous ridges with oral implants. *Clinical Oral Implants Research*, Vol.17, Suppl 2, (October 2006), pp. 136-159, ISSN 0905-7161

Chiapasco, M., Zaniboni, M. & Rimondini, L. (2007) Autogenous onlay bone grafts vs. alveolar distraction osteogenesis for the correction of vertically deficient edentulous ridges: a 2-4-year prospective study on humans. *Clinical Oral Implants Research*, Vol.18, No.4, (August 2007), pp. 432-440, ISSN 0905-7161

Chiapasco, M., Zaniboni, M. & Rimondini, L. (2008) Dental implants placed in grafted maxillary sinuses: a retrospective analysis of clinical outcome according to the initial clinical situation and a proposal of defect classification. *Clinical Oral Implants Research*, Vol.19, No.4, (April 2008), pp. 416-428, ISSN 0905-7161

Chiapasco, M., Casentini, P. & Zaniboni, M. (2009) Bone augmentation procedures in implant dentistry. *The International Journal of Oral & Maxillofacial Implants*, Vol.24, Suppl, (October 2009), pp. 237-259, ISSN 0882-2786

Chrcanovic, B.R. & Custódio, A.L. (2009) Inferior alveolar nerve lateral transposition. *Oral and Maxillofacial Surgery,*. Vol.13, No.4, (December 2009), pp.213-219, ISSN 1865-1550

Danza, M., Guidi, R. & Carinci, F. (2009) Comparison between implants inserted into piezo split and unsplit alveolar crests. *Journal of Oral and Maxillofacial Surgery*, Vol.67, No.11, (November 2009), pp. 2460-2465, ISSN 0278-2391

das Neves, F.D., Fones, D., Bernardes, S.R., do Prado, C.J. & Neto, A.J. (2006) Short implants - an analysis of longitudinal studies. *The International Journal of Oral & Maxillofacial Implants*, Vol.21, No.1, (January 2006), pp. 86-93, ISSN 0882-2786

Del Fabbro, M., Bellini, C.M., Romeo, D. & Francetti, L. (2011) Tilted Implants for the Rehabilitation of Edentulous Jaws: A Systematic Review. *Clinical Implant Dentistry and Related Research*, Epub ahead of print, ISSN 1708-8208

Donos, N., Mardas, N. & Chadha, V. (2008) Clinical outcomes of implants following lateral bone augmentation: systematic assessment of available options (barrier membranes, bone grafts, split osteotomy). *Journal of Clinical Periodontology*, Vol.35, Suppl, (September 2008), pp. 173-202, ISSN 0303-6979

Emmerich, D., Att, W. & Stappert, C. (2005) Sinus floor elevation using osteotomes: a systematic review and meta-analysis. *Journal of Periodontology*, Vol.76, No.8, (August 2005), pp. 1237-1251, ISSN 0022-3492

Esposito, M., Worthington, H.V. & Coulthard, P. (2005) Interventions for replacing missing teeth: dental implants in zygomatic bone for the rehabilitation of the severely deficient edentulous maxilla. *Cochrane Database of Systematic Reviews*, Vol.19, No.4, (October 2005), CD004151, ISSN 1469-493X

Esposito, M., Grusovin, M.G., Felice, P., Karatzopoulos, G., Worthington, H.V. & Coulthard, P. (2009) Interventions for replacing missing teeth: horizontal and vertical bone augmentation techniques for dental implant treatment. *Cochrane Database of Systematic Reviews*, Vol.7, No.4, (October 2009), CD003607, ISSN 1469-493X

Esposito, M., Grusovin, M.G., Rees, J., Karasoulos, D., Felice, P., Alissa, R., Worthington, H.V. & Coulthard, P. (2010) Interventions for replacing missing teeth: augmentation procedures of the maxillary sinus. *Cochrane Database of Systematic Reviews*, Vol.17, No.3, (March 2010), CD008397, ISSN 1469-493

Esposito, M., Pellegrino, G., Pistilli, R. & Felice, P. (2011) Rehabilitation of postrior atrophic edentulous jaws: prostheses supported by 5 mm short implants or by longer implants in augmented bone? One-year results from a pilot randomised clinical trial. *European Journal of Oral* Implantology, Vol.4, No.1, (Spring 2011), pp. 21-30, ISSN 1756-2406

Felice, P., Cannizzaro, G., Checchi, V., Marchetti, C., Pellegrino, G., Censi, P. & Esposito, M. (2009) Vertical bone augmentation versus 7-mm-long implants in posterior atrophic mandibles. Results of a randomised controlled clinical trial of up to 4 months after loading. European Journal of Oral Implantology, Vol.2, No.1, (Spring 2009), pp. 7-20, ISSN 1756-2406

Felice, P., Pellegrino, G., Checchi, L., Pistilli, R. & Esposito, M. (2010) Vertical augmentation with interpositional blocks of anorganic bovine bone vs. 7-mm-long implants in posterior mandibles: 1-year results of a randomized clinical trial. *Clinical Oral Implants Research*, Vol.21, No.12, (December 2010), pp. 1394-1403, ISSN 0905-7161

Friberg, B. (2008) The posterior maxilla: clinical considerations and current concepts using Brånemark System implants. *Periodontology 2000*, Vol.47, No.1, (June 2008), pp. 67-78, ISSN 0906-6713

Flemmig, T.F. & Beikler, T. (2009) Decision making in implant dentistry: an evidence-based and decision-analysis approach. *Periodontology 2000*, Vol.50, No.1, (June 2009), pp. 154-172, ISSN 0906-6713

Gabbert, O., Koob, A., Schmitter, M. & Rammelsberg, P. (2009) Implants placed in combination with an internal sinus lift without graft material: an analysis of short-term failure. *Journal of Clinical Periodontology*, Vol.36, No.2, (February 2009), pp. 177-183, ISSN 0303-6979

Graziani, F., Donos, N., Needleman, I., Gabriele, M. & Tonetti, M. (2004) Comparison of implant survival following sinus floor augmentation procedures with implants placed in pristine posterior maxillary bone: a systematic review. *Clinical Oral Implants Research*, Vol.15, No.6, (December 2004), pp. 677-682, ISSN 0905-7161

Griffin, T.J. & Cheung, W.S. (2004) The use of short, wide implants in posterior areas with reduced bone height: a retrospective investigation. *The Journal of Prosthetic Dentistry*, Vol.92, No.2, (August 2004), pp. 139-144, ISSN 0022-3913

Guyatt, G.H., Oxman, A.D., Schünemann, H.J., Tugwell, P. & Knottnerus, A. (2011) GRADE guidelines: a new series of articles in the Journal of Clinical Epidemiology. *Journal of Clinical Epidemiology*, Vol.64, No.4, (April 2011), pp. 380-382, ISSN 0895-4356

Hagi, D., Deporter, D.A., Pilliar, R.M. & Arenovich, T. (2004) A targeted review of study outcomes with short (< or = 7 mm) endosseous dental implants placed in partially edentulous patients. *Journal of Periodontology*, Vol.75, No.6, (June 2004), pp. 798-804, ISSN 0022-3492

Holtzclaw, D.J., Toscano, N.J. & Rosen, P.S. (2010) Reconstruction of posterior mandibular alveolar ridge deficiencies with the piezoelectric hinge-assisted ridge split technique: a retrospective observational report. *Journal of Periodontology*, Vol.81, No.11, (November 2010), pp. 1580-1586, ISSN 0022-3492

Howick, J., Chalmers, I., Glasziou, P., Greenhalgh, T., Heneghan, C., Liberati, A., Moschetti, I., Phillips, B., Thornton, H., Goddard, O. & Hodgkinson, M. (2011). The Oxford 2011 Levels of Evidence, Oxford Centre for Evidence-Based Medicine, 01.08.2011, Available from http://www.cebm.net/index.aspx?o=5653

Jensen, O.T., Cockrell, R., Kuhike, L. & Reed, C. (2002) Anterior maxillary alveolar distraction osteogenesis: a prospective 5-year clinical study. *The International Journal of Oral & Maxillofacial Implants*, Vol.17, No.1, (January 2002), pp. 52-68, ISSN 0882-2786

Jensen, O.T., Cullum, D.R. & Baer, D. (2009) Marginal bone stability using 3 different flap approaches for alveolar split expansion for dental implants: a 1-year clinical study. *Journal of Oral and Maxillofacial Surgery*, Vol.67, No.9, (September 2009), pp. 1921-1930, ISSN 0278-2391

Jensen, S.S. & Terheyden, H. (2009) Bone augmentation procedures in localized defects in the alveolar ridge: clinical results with different bone grafts and bone-substitute materials. *The International Journal of Oral & Maxillofacial Implants*, Vol.24, Suppl, (October 2009), pp. 218-236, ISSN 0882-2786

Jung, R.E., Schneider, D., Ganeles, J., Wismeijer, D., Zwahlen, M., Hämmerle, C.H. & Tahmaseb, A. (2009) Computer technology applications in surgical implant dentistry: a systematic review. *The International Journal of Oral & Maxillofacial Implants*, Vol.24, Suppl, (October 2009), pp. 92-109, ISSN 0882-2786

Keller, E.E. (1995) Reconstruction of the severely atrophic edentulous mandible with endosseous implants: a 10-year longitudinal study. *Journal of Oral and Maxillofacial Surgery*, Vol.53, No.3, (March 1995), pp. 305-320, ISSN 0278-2391

Kotsovilis, S., Fourmousis, I., Karoussis, I.K. & Bamia, C. (2009) A systematic review and meta-analysis on the effect of implant length on the survival of rough-surface dental implants. *Journal of Periodontology*, Vol.80, No.11, (November 2009), pp. 1700-1718, ISSN 0022-3492

Lundgren, S., Moy, P., Johansson, C. & Nilsson, H. (1996) Augmentation of the maxillary sinus floor with particulated mandible: a histologic and histomorphometric study. *The International Journal of Oral & Maxillofacial Implants*, Vol.11, No.6, (November 1996), pp. 760-766, ISSN 0882-2786

Lundgren, S., Sjöström, M., Nyström, E. & Sennerby, L. (2008) Strategies in reconstruction of the atrophic maxilla with autogenous bone grafts and endosseous implants. *Periodontology 2000*, Vol.47, No.1, (June 2008), pp. 143-161, ISSN 0906-6713

Maló, P., de Araújo Nobre, M. & Rangert, B. (2007) Short implants placed one-stage in maxillae and mandibles: a retrospective clinical study with 1 to 9 years of follow-up. *Clinical Implant Dentistry and Related Research*, Vol.9, No.1, (March 2007), pp. 15-21, ISSN 1523-0899

Meijndert, L., Raghoebar, G.M., Schüpbach, P., Meijer, H.J. & Vissink, A. (2005) Bone quality at the implant site after reconstruction of a local defect of the maxillary anterior ridge with chin bone or deproteinised cancellous bovine bone. *International Journal of Oral and Maxillofacial Surgery*, Vol.34, No.8, (December 2005), pp. 877-884, ISSN 0901-5027

Meijndert, L., Meijer, H.J., Stellingsma, K., Stegenga, B. & Raghoebar, G.M. (2007) Evaluation of aesthetics of implant-supported single-tooth replacements using different bone augmentation procedures: a prospective randomized clinical study. *Clinical Oral Implants Research*, Vol.18, No.6, (December 2007), pp. 715-719, ISSN 0905-7161

Özkan, Y., Özcan, M., Varol, A., Akoglu, B., Ucankale, M. & Basa, S. (2007) Resonance frequency analysis assessment of implant stability in labial onlay grafted posterior mandibles: a pilot clinical study. *The International Journal of Oral & Maxillofacial Implants*, Vol.22, No.2, (March 2007), pp. 235-242, ISSN 0882-2786

Pjetursson, B.E., Tan, W.C., Zwahlen, M. & Lang, N.P. (2008) A systematic review of the success of sinus floor elevation and survival of implants inserted in combination with sinus floor elevation. *Journal of Clinical Periodontology*, Vol.35, Suppl, (September 2008), pp. 216-240, ISSN 0303-6979

Pommer, B., Unger, E., Sütö, D., Hack, N. & Watzek, G. (2009) Mechanical properties of the Schneiderian membrane in vitro. *Clinical Oral Implants Research*, Vol.20, No.6, (June 2009), pp. 633-637, ISSN 0905-7161

Pommer, B. & Watzek, G. (2009) Gel-pressure technique for flapless transcrestal maxillary sinus floor elevation: a preliminary cadaveric study of a new surgical technique. *The International Journal of Oral & Maxillofacial Implants*, Vol.24, No.5, (September 2009), pp. 817-822, ISSN 0882-2786

Pommer, B., Frantal, S., Willer, J., Posch, M., Watzek, G. & Tepper, G. (2011) Impact of dental implant length on early failure rates: a meta-analysis of observational studies. *Journal of Clinical Periodontology*, Vol.38, No.9, (September 2011), pp. 856-863, ISSN 0303-6979

Raghoebar, G.M., den Hartog, L. & Vissink, A. (2010) Augmentation in proximity to the incisive foramen to allow placement of endosseous implants: a case series. *Journal of Oral and Maxillofacial Surgery*, Vol.68, No.9, (September 2009), pp. 2267-2271, ISSN 0278-2391

Renouard, F. & Nisand, D. (2006) Impact of implant length and diameter on survival rates. *Clinical Oral Implants Research*, Vol.17, Suppl 2, (October 2006), pp. 35-51, ISSN 0905-7161

Rocchietta, I., Fontana, F. & Simion, M. (2008) Clinical outcomes of vertical bone augmentation to enable dental implant placement: a systematic review. *Journal of Clinical Periodontology*, Vol.35, Suppl, (September 2008), pp. 203-215, ISSN 0303-6979

Sbordone, L., Toti, P., Menchini-Fabris, G., Sbordone, C. & Guidetti, F. (2009) Implant survival in maxillary and mandibular osseous onlay grafts and native bone: a 3-year clinical and computerized tomographic follow-up. *The International Journal of Oral & Maxillofacial Implants*, Vol.24, No.4, (July 2009), pp. 695-703, ISSN 0882-2786

Seibert, J.S. (1983) Reconstruction of deformed, partially edentulous ridges, using full thickness onlay grafts. Part I. Technique and wound healing. *Compendium of Continuing Education in Dentistry*, Vol.4, No.5, (September 1983), pp. 437-453, ISSN 1548-8578

Sjöström, M., Lundgren, S. & Sennerby, L. (2006) A histomorphometric comparison of the bone graft-titanium interface between interpositional and onlay/inlay bone grafting techniques. *The International Journal of Oral & Maxillofacial Implants*, Vol.21, No.1, (January 2006), pp. 52-62, ISSN 0882-2786

Slade, G.D. & Spencer, A.J. (1994) Development and evaluation of the Oral Health Impact Profile. *Community Dental Health*, Vol.11, No.1, (March 1994), pp. 3-11, ISSN 0265-539X

Sohn, D.S., Lee, H.J., Heo, J.U., Moon, J.W., Park, I.S. & Romanos, G.E. (2010) Immediate and delayed lateral ridge expansion technique in the atrophic posterior mandibular ridge. *Journal of Oral and Maxillofacial Surgery*, Vol.68, No.9, (September 2010), pp. 2283-2290, ISSN 0278-2391

Stellingsma, K., Bouma, J., Stegenga, B., Meijer, H.J. & Raghoebar, G.M. (2003) Satisfaction and psychosocial aspects of patients with an extremely resorbed mandible treated with implant-retained overdentures. A prospective, comparative study. *Clinical Oral Implants Research*, Vol.14, No.2, (April 2003), pp. 166-172, ISSN 0905-7161

Stellingsma, C., Vissink, A., Meijer, H.J., Kuiper, C. & Raghoebar, G.M. (2004) Implantology and the severely resorbed edentulous mandible. *Critical Reviews in Oral Biology and Medicine*, Vol.15, No.4, (July 2004), pp. 240-248, ISSN 1045-4411

Tan, W.C., Lang, N.P., Zwahlen, M. & Pjetursson, B.E. (2008) A systematic review of the success of sinus floor elevation and survival of implants inserted in combination with sinus floor elevation. Part II: transalveolar technique. *Journal of Clinical Periodontology*, Vol.35, Suppl, (September 2008), pp. 241-254, ISSN 0303-6979

Vasak, C., Watzak, G., Gahleitner, A., Strbac, G., Schemper, M. & Zechner, W. (2011) Computed tomography-based evaluation of template (NobelGuide™)-guided implant positions: a prospective radiological study. *Clinical Oral Implants Research*, Epub ahead of print, ISSN 1600-0501

Waasdorp, J. & Reynolds, M.A. (2010) Allogeneic bone onlay grafts for alveolar ridge augmentation: a systematic review. *The International Journal of Oral & Maxillofacial Implants*, Vol.25, No.3, (May 2010), pp. 525-531, ISSN 0882-2786

Wiltfang, J., Schultze-Mosgau, S., Nkenke, E., Thorwarth, M., Neukam, F.W. & Schlegel, K.A. (2005) Onlay augmentation versus sinuslift procedure in the treatment of severely resorbed maxilla: a 5-year comparative longitudinal study. *International Journal of Oral and Maxillofacial Surgery*, Vol.34, No.8, (December 2005), pp. 885-889, ISSN 0901-5027

Zitzmann, N.U. & Schärer, P. (1998) Sinus elevation procedures in the resorbed posterior maxilla. Comparison of the crestal and lateral approaches. *Oral Surgery, Oral Medicine, Oral Pathology, Oral Radiology, and Endodontics*, Vol.85, No.1, (January 1998), pp. 8-17, ISSN 1079-2104

Zitzmann, N.U., Schärer, P. & Marinello, C.P. (2001) Long-term results of implants treated with guided bone regeneration: a 5-year prospective study. *The International Journal of Oral & Maxillofacial Implants*, Vol.16, No.3, (May 2001), pp. 355-366, ISSN 0882-2786

12

Clinical Concepts in Oral and Maxillofacial Surgery and Novel Findings to the Field of Bone Regeneration

Annika Rosén and Rachael Sugars
Div of Oral and Maxillofacial Surgery and the Craniofacial Stem Cell Biology Group,
Div of Oral Biology, Dept. of Dental Medicine, Karolinska Institutet, Huddinge,
Sweden

1. Introduction

In an increasingly aging population, where aesthetics plays an important role in society, the loss of bone and teeth due to disease or trauma places a large burden on healthcare systems worldwide. It is estimated that more than 2.2 million grafting procedures are performed annually to repair bone defects in orthopedics, neurosurgery and dentistry (Giannoudis et al, 2005). Following surgical intervention the use of bone grafts / substitute materials or distraction osteogenesis (DO) for the expansion of the maxialla are current approaches to facilitate bone regeneration. What is regeneration and how is it defined? Regeneration can be defined as "the reproduction or reconstruction of a lost or injured part of the body in such a way that the architecture and function of the lost or injured tissues are completely restored" (Bosshardt et al, 2009), and as such it is necessary to consider the cells that are involved to produce the destroyed tissues, how can these cells be stimulated and is a space filler required to support the cells and to hold signaling molecules? Bone formation is a complex and dynamic process involving the interactions between cells and the surrounding milieu. Repair occurs before regeneration but where healing occurs first without restoration of function. The current chapter considers clinical approaches, cases and requirements for bone regeneration and brings it together with a biological perspective of the cellular and biomolecular interactions necessary to stimulate new bone formation. Given the increasing need for grafting procedures and the limitations to current grafting techniques the future applications of tissue engineering approaches are finally discussed.

2. Clinical applications

Reconstructive surgery for bony defects in the oral and maxillofacial region is a challenge. The gold standard for reconstructive surgery remains autogenous bone grafting that is osteoconductive and osteoinductive, and from an immunological point of view safe. Donor sites are available either intra- or extra orally. The intraoral harvesting sites are in the maxillary tuberosity and in the mandibular ramus, retromandibular area and the symphysis. The bone is often of cortical nature and the volume limited. Harvesting can be performed during local anesthesia often in combination with sedation. Harvesting bone from extra-oral sites is required when larger amounts are required. The iliac crest, tibia, costochondral bone or calvarium bone are common donor sites but general anesthesia and hospitalization of the patient is needed. The bone is both of cortical and cancellous/trabecular nature. When it is not possible to harvest bone due to the patient's medical history or limited resources, DO, a relatively new technique in the field of oral and maxillofacial surgery has been developed. This technique has also been useful in reconstructive surgery for genetic anomalies.

2.1 Reconstruction of resorbed alveolar crests

Edentulous severely resorbed maxillas are a major problem for patients when prosthodontic treatment and dental implants are necessary. The standard procedure installs the implants vertically in the alveolar crest with the implant totally covered by bone. The bone volume needs to be at least 10 mm in the vertical dimension and 4 mm in the horizontal aspect in the maxillary alveolar crest with this technique. In patients with less bone volume bone grafting is an alternative. Tilted implants were first presented by Mattsson and colleagues as an alternative method to bone grafting in severely resorbed alveolar crest, classes V and VI (Mattson et al 1999). The method of tilting the implants was used to reach the maximum length of the prosthodontic bridge. Recently, we presented a 10-year follow-up study on patients treated with this technique. The success rate was 97 % (Rosén et al 2007). One reason for the high success rate could be attributed to the use of longer implants, thereby improving the anchorage in dense bone compared to conventional implant treatments. Another advantage was that the prosthetic construction could be more posteriorly directed in the arch and result in the equalisation of loading across the bridge. Krekmanow and collaborators have reported biomechanical measurements in tilting implants, which showed no negative effects on load distribution in the fixed prosthesis constructions (Krekmanow et al 2000). Furthermore, the method by which implants are tilted is relatively easy for the surgeon to perform and reduces the patient's treatment time (Fig. 1).

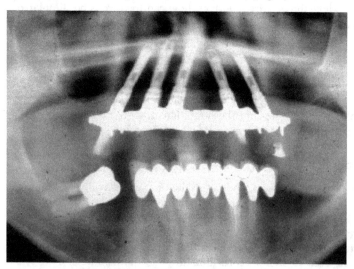

Fig. 1. X-ray, patient treated with tilted implants.

2.2 Sinus lift

The first use of bone grafting to the maxillary sinus was presented in the 1960s by Boyne (Boyne 1969). He performed a so-called Caldwell-Luc opening, where a fenestration of the bone to the maxillary sinus made it possible to elevate the sinus membrane. Autogenous bone and marrow grafts were placed on the sinus floor. Approximately three months after surgery an increase of osseous tissue was seen. In a review by Triplett and collegues (Triplett et al 2000), they described the material choices for sinus augmentation, and concluded that autogenous bone was the best choice as it was osteoinductive, osteoconductive and contained osteoblasts and osteoprogenitor cells. The technique of sinus grafting has been used for placement of dental implants since then.

Sinus lift with an osteotom is another even easier technique to perform, when maxilla bone is moderately resorbed. The technique involves a series of increasingly wide osteotomes, which allows site preparation for the implant while also expanding the apical portion of the alveolus into the sinus. The elevated sinus membrane remains intact and bone forms beneath the elevated membrane, commonly 3-4 mm of floor height is effectively gained. The bone cells migrate from both the base of the sinus maxillaries and from the bone chip that is uplifted into the sinus. From the start the bone height has to be at least 4 mm so that a 9 or 11 mm implant can be installed. The concept of "tenting-up" the membrane in both the sinus floor and the nasal floor was first described by Brånemark (Brånemark et al 1984).

A 2-3-year follow-up study evaluated the survival rate of dental implants placed in partially or totally edentulous maxillae, with moderately resorbed bone (Dabirian and Rosén 2004). The implants were placed directly in the bone of the maxillae or in bone graft sites in sinus maxillaries using the sinus lift technique with an osteotom. The number of healthy patients treated with implants in the study was 126. The total number of implants was 232, 1 - 6 implants in each patient. Each patient was examined yearly with oral inspection and x-ray. The follow-up period was 2 - 4 years (mean of 3 years). The results showed satisfactory implant survival rates of 99.6 % after at least 2 years of clinical function. Only one implant was reported to have failed. However, in the radiological examinations, marginal bone loss of greater than 0.2 mm per year was observed in 22.8 % of the cases. The study showed that maxillary sinus floor grafting could be performed where the maxillary bone does not offer adequate space for the implants without affecting the survival rate of these implants.

2.3 Bone grafting

Bone grafting is a frequently used method where autogenous bone is transplanted to defected jaws (Nyström et al 2004). The harvested bone can be placed as inlays or onlays both in the maxilla and in the mandible. Inlay means when the bone is placed inside, for example in the sinus maxillaries as a bone chip, particulate bone or in between two bony fragments. Onlay means when a bone block is fixed with titanium plates and screws on the buccal or lingual part of the alveolar ridge. However, bone grafting is time- consuming due to the extra time needed for the graft to augment until time for dental implant installation, typically 6 months. After the grafting procedure, the bone block becomes almost necrotic and will be incorporated by revascularization induced by the inflammatory reaction during the first week after implantation, the healing phase. In the case of cancellous particulate bone grafts, which have a larger surface area than the bone block, vascularization from the surrounding tissue occurs faster. It is incorporated quicker but there is also the risk of a faster resorption. Grafting will often necessitate general anesthesia and hospitalisation, which is costly to national healthcare systems. Despite the high success rate for the tilted implant procedure, today the gold standard is still autogenous bone grafts; not only for implant treatment but for all kinds of osseous defects in oral and maxillofacial regions. One side effect is that the bone cannot be expanded in the vertical height when using the onlay technique, only in the horizontal dimension which makes the alveolar crest wider so there is enough space for the implants. The inlay technique, however, can expand the alveolar bone in the vertical dimension in the maxilla. A Le Fort I osteotomy is used to expand the space for the transplanted autogenous bone and stabilization of the transplanted bone is made by titanium plates and screws (Fig. 2).

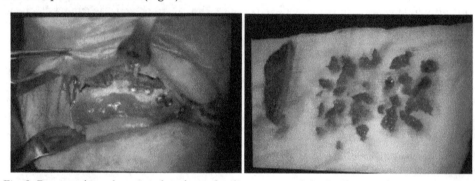

Fig. 2. Bone grafting, bone is taken from the iliac crest, and the Le Fort I technique is used to expand the vertical height in the maxilla.

This technique can be useful when the sagital dimension is not optimal for dental implant treatment. With the Le Fort I osteotomy the maxilla can be moved forward for optimal occlusion. Side effects, such as postoperative problems with the graft or host site morbidity can be observed as well as resorption of the bone if an extended healing time is required. It is very important to cover the osteotomy with a tension free flap otherwise, a gap in the incision area will be the result and the chances of an infection or the resorption of the transplanted bone increases. These surgical procedures also entail some risks in the form of nerve damage (Kahnberg, 2010).

2.4 Synthetic bone building technique

Bone-building therapies, such as synthetic bone, allogenic, or bone from different species, xenogenic, have been used extensively in the past with satisfactory results. However, the healing time for biomaterial grafts is longer than for autogenous bone and it may also give rise to rejection and infection. Rejection of the bone or possible transmission of infections from these types of bone-building therapies is a danger (Maiorana, 2010).

2.5 Distraction osteogenesis

Distraction osteogenesis (DO) is a method for either restoring atrophic jaws in the vertical dimension or for expanding congenital defected jaws in the orofacial region (Cheung et al 2010). DO is a clinical tissue engineering method with huge possibilities, even to treat severe deformities in the craniofacial area. Patients with hemi-facial asymmetries, extreme retrognatic maxillas or mandibles can be adjusted to normal positions. The device can be intra- or extraorally fixated with titanium screws in the bone. The major advantages are that bone grafts are not necessary and the technique allowing the soft tissue to expand in the oral region. The technique consists of five phases, the osteotomy, the latency, active distractor, consolidation and remodeling. The osteotomy triggers a biological process of bone repair. A blood clot appears and will be replaced by granulation tissue which consists of inflammation cells. Fibroblasts, collagen and invading capillaries fill the distracted bone space and stimulate the osteocytes. This technique can even be used in temporomandibular joint (TMJ) reconstruction, in cases with ankylosis where the condyle is resected. The TMJ distraction creates a neocondyle in the bone of ramus mandibulae, the bone moves gradually towards the glenoid fossa and the normal anatomical structures will be restored. Long term stability of the TMJ has been reported (Cheung et al 2007).

DO is a two-stage surgical technique and can be used when teeth are missing and the alveolar ridge needs to be vertically expanded with bone before dental implants are placed (Cano et al 2006) or in the cases of an open bite with good occlusion in the molar region of the jaws when conventional orthognathic surgery is not an alternative. A reliable patient is needed who must expand the device each day and it also necessitates a long retaining period including orthodontic treatment. After the retaining period the device has to be removed surgically. Infections, bone morbidity and distracter fractures are side effects that have been reported (Saulacic et al 2009).

Recently, two patient cases in our clinic with open bite and normal occlusion in the premolar and molar region were treated with the osteodistraction technique. Patient 1, a 22-year old male with a three-year follow-up and patient 2, a 40-year old female with a two-year follow-up were treated. The alveolar ridge was vertically expanded in the frontal maxillary area in both cases. The intra orally distraction devises were surgical inserted under general anesthesia (Fig. 3).

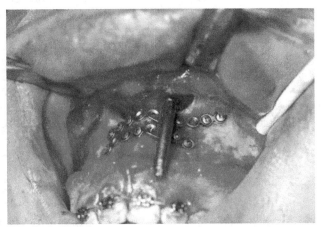

Fig. 3. The distraction device surgically inserted in the frontal maxilla in patient 1.

After a couple of nights in hospital the patients went home and after approximately one week they were instructed to do the expansion two times a day. After three to four weeks the maxillary frontal regions were expanded to a normal occlusion. The orthodontic treatment started whilst the distraction device remained for a three month retaining phase. After a year, the orthodontic treatments were finished and good results were obtained in both patients. The patients were satisfied with the results and no side effects were seen (Fig. 4).

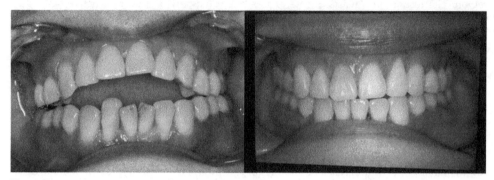

Fig. 4. Pre- and postoperative close up pictures of patient 2 with an open bite and treated with DO.

Patient 1 developed a necrotic tooth pulp after two years, which had to be endodontically treated, probably a side effect of the orthodontic treatment. A three year follow-up study will soon be reported (Rosén et al in manuscript).

2.6 Surgically assisted rapid maxillary expansion (Sarme)

Orthopedic maxillary expansion (OME) is a common method used in children for treating uni- or bilateral cross bites, cleft lip and palate, and patients with maxillary teeth crowding to gain arch length. In teenage children or in adults where the bone is mature and therefore harder, limited expansion occurs only with dental changes. Surgical procedures such as Le Fort I osteotomy for widening the maxilla in a transverse dimension has been an alternative to OME in teenage children and for adults. The combined surgical and orthodontic treatment for maxillary expansion with only tooth anchorage often show post retention relapses with the Hyrax-type expander. Several types of surgical assisted rapid maxillary expansion (SARME) devices with bone anchorage have thereafter been presented, the transversal palatinal Surgi-Tec, the Rotterdam Palatal distracter, the Magdeburg palatal distracter and the Smile distracter. Recently, a three year follow-up study was reported where OME or SARME were compared with a control group. The control group consisted of untreated, skeletal Class 1 subjects matched to the OME group in order to assess the effects of normal skeletal growth. The study showed that both the OME and the SARME procedures remained stable after three years with some amount of post retention relapses compared with the control group (Kurt et al 2010). In our clinic, we went one step further using a device with both tooth and bone anchorages (Fig. 6). A long time follow-up study of this technique will soon be presented. The study included 43 patients treated with the tooth and bone anchored device. Palatinal expansion up to 15 mm occurred, in patients where the canines had supra position and no space at all in the arch (Rosén et al, in manuscript).

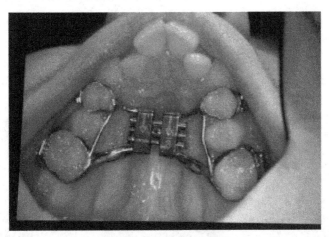

Fig. 6. A SARME device with both teeth and bone anchorages. Palatinal screws are hidden on each side under the posterior part of the device

2.7 Osteogenesis imperfecta

Osteogenesis imperfecta (OI) is an inherited genetic disorder. The connective tissues are affected throughout the whole body, including the dentin of the teeth. To date, seven types of OI have been identified varying from the mild Type I OI to the moderate Types IV and VI, severe Types III, V and VII to lethal Type II (Martin and Shapiro, 2007). Multiple fractures of long bones are frequently observed as well as disturbances of the permanent dentition. Orthognathic surgery in patients with OI is rare but necessary to correct the malocclusion for functional and esthetic reasons. Most cases result in a successful outcome with stable and good dental occlusion. Two patients probably with severe types I and IV OI, and malocclusion class III with retrognathic maxilla and prognathic mandible, were treated with orthodontic treatment and bimaxillary surgical correction (Rosén et al 2011).

Patient 1, a 26-year old male with most likely OI type IV was treated. Since childhood he had been treated for 18 fractures of the limbs and hips. The analysis indicated advancement of 8 mm of the maxilla and a setback mandible of 4 mm. The surgical procedure was planned with certain precautions with a two step model. Firstly, a Le Fort I osteotomy where a stable occlusion was planned for so the surgery could be interrupted in case the bone was too brittle. Secondly, a setback vertical ramus osteotomy followed by an intermaxillary fixation for five weeks. We tested the bone in the maxilla with titanium screws before any osteotomies were performed to ensure their function in the soft bone before continuation. We planned to use wires or a halo frame for stabilization if the bone proved to be too soft. The surgical outcome in patient 1 was good and the surgery was made in one session. The maxillary bone was thin and teeth were brittle but the orthodontic anchorage was stable enough to fixate the jaws together and the titanium screws remained stable in the bone when the titanium plates were fixed over the osteotomies.

Case 2, a 22-year old male with OI severe type I was planned for a 10 mm advancement of the maxilla with a Le Fort I osteotomy and 6-7 mm set back with a vertical ramus osteotomy of the mandible. A bone graft from the iliac crest was planned if necessary. However, there was no need for bone graft during surgery and the operation followed a routine fashion and was completed after five weeks of intermaxillary fixation. We concluded that it was possible to perform combined orthodontic and orthognathic surgery in patients with OI despite the greater risk of complications such as fractures in the soft bone and loss of orthodontic anchorage in brittle teeth. The treatments were successful in both cases with follow-up times of five to six years (Fig. 7, Rosén et al 2011).

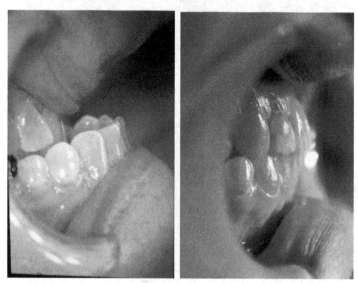

Fig. 7 a and b. Surgically treated patient with OI. The patient no. 1 underwent bimaxillary surgery and the profile photos are pre-and postoperative.

3. Biological considerations

The dynamic interplay between the cells and the environment is essential to ensure successful bone formation and regeneration, a feature easily forgotten during the establishment of new clinical strategies. Therefore to fully understand bone grafting and regeneration an appreciation of bone mineralization, and the interplay with the biochemical environment is necessary. In many cases after maxillofacial surgery, wound healing occurs before new bone is deposited. Bone formation is a carefully balanced process involving the secretion of an organic pre-mineralized matrix, osteoid, that becomes mineralized with inorganic hydroxyapaptite (HAP) crystals and its subsequent resorption and remodeling. The interactions with the surrounding biochemical milieu stimulate cell migration, adhesion, proliferation, differentiation, transcription and translation. Resulting in the synthesis and secretion of an extracellular matrix (ECM) that acts as a scaffold for mineral deposition and nucleation, and serves to sequester and protect growth factors.

3.1 Wound healing

Wound healing is a unique and complex system, where the healing of both soft and hard tissues needs to be fully integrated. For this to occur a coordinated series of events must be induced, i) stimulation of an initial inflammatory response, ii) the recruitment of specific cell types and iii) induction of their proliferation leading to bone formation. A model has been devised for wound healing in the epithelia but it is also relevant in this context, particularly with DO (Wikesjsö et al, 2010). Initially, clots form followed by early stages of inflammation with the infiltration of inflammatory cells, such as neutorphils and monocytes into the clot. This takes place just hours after damage and cleanses the wound of bacteria and necrotic debris. After a few days, the late phase of inflammation is initiated along with macrophages infiltrating into the wound. Macrophages assist the formation of granulation tissue and the release of growth factors that stimulate fibroblasts. The granulation tissue matures becoming rich in cells and the collagen-rich ECM provides a suitable environment for further cell propagation and reconstruction of the vasculature prior to bone formation.

3.2 Bone formation

Bone formation occurs by two distinct condensation processes; endochondral, which forms the long bones and intramembraneous that results in the flat bones of the jaws and calvaria. Endochondral bone formation occurs when mesenchymal stem cells (MSCs) migrate and condensate at a high density at regions where skeletal rudiments will develop. MSCs differentiate into chondrocytes to form an avascular anlagen, into which they secrete an ECM rich in type II collagen and aggrecan, and express typical chondrocytic transcription factors, such as Sox 5/6/9. As proliferation ceases, the epiphyseal growth plate begins to form with the cells becoming hypertrophic, synthesizing type X collagen and blood vessels finally penetrate into the cartilage template. The hypertrophic chondrocytes undergo apoptosis and are replaced by osteoblasts recruited from the perichondrium to form the bone collar and together with bone elongation create the bone marrow space. In comparison, intramembraneous ossification results from the direct condensation and differentiation of MSCs into osteoblasts in regions that are rich in blood vessels. The resulting woven or primary bone forms rapidly, particularly during embryogenesis, in the case of DO, after fracture healing and during adaptive bone gain after mechanical loading. Despite these two distinct formation pathways both types of bone share some common molecular and cellular control mechanisms.

3.3 Bone cell differentiation

Biomineralization is a dynamic process driven by active osteoblasts that initially secrete an osteoid that eventually becomes mineralized. The mature cells are polarized and cuboidal, a proportion of which are termed bone-lining cells and become flattened and align along the bone surface. Whereas the remainder become entrapped and embedded within the forming mineralized tissue within the lacunae of the matrix called osteocytes. The precise function of osteocytes remains to be clarified however evidence suggests that the cells have a role in response to mechanical stimuli, as a mechanoreceptor (Aarden et al, 1994).

Osteoblast progenitors are derived from MSCs, which originate as pericytes along the blood vessels within the bone marrow in a niche that is finely balanced with hematopoiesis (Bianco et al, 2011). MSC differentiation gives rise to a number of different lineages that acquire specific phenotypes under the control of specific regulatory factors. Characterization of the osteoblast differentiation process has been defined into three stages; a growth or proliferation stage, matrix maturation stage and mineralization stage. During the first phase of growth and proliferation the cells exhibit high mitotic activity and actively express cell-cycle associated genes. At this time ECM associated molecules are synthesized including collagen type I, osteopontin (OPN) and fibronectin. Collagen type I continues to be expressed with proliferation but at low levels whereas the other ECM proteins are all down-regulated. As the cells move into the second stage of matrix maturation, alkaline phosphate levels dramatically increase and there is considerable secretion and organization of the organic ECM in preparation for the final phase of mineralization and the deposition of HAP crystals. The secreted ECM molecules play a considerable role in this dynamic process, including collagen type I, glycoproteins, sialoproteins and proteoglycans, and their roles will be discussed in more detail below.

Each of the phases of osteoblast differentiation is characterized by a set of specific genes and regulatory molecules that allow progression into the next stage (Marie, 2008). The initial and key transcription factor is Runx2, also known as Core-binding factor alpha 1, a member of the Runt-related factors (Runx) family of transcription factors. Runx2 activates vital bone ECM genes, including collagen type 1 alpha 1 (COL1A1) and osteocalcin (OCN). It is important to note that Runx2 is also expressed by cells other than osteoblasts, including chondrocytes, T-cells and other mesenchymal cells. However, two separate promoters have been identified; an upstream promoter that specifically drives the expression of osteoblast-specific isoforms, whereas the downstream promoter activates Runx2 isoforms in T-cells, although some expression has been identified in osteoblasts (Harada et al, 1999). Runx2 is essential for both endochondral and intramembraneous bone formation, as targeted disruption of the gene results in a complete lack of bone formation in both processes (Komori et al, 1997). On the other hand, over expression of Runx2, such as by skin fibroblasts, which do not normally express the molecule, exhibit osteoblast-specific gene expression (Takeda et al, 2001). In addition to being the initiator of osteoblast differentiation, it functions as an inhibitor of progenitor proliferation and is required for terminally differentiated osteoblast function. Downstream of Runx2, osterix (OSX, Sp7), a zinc-finger-containing transcription factor and bone morphogenic protein (BMP) 2-inducible gene has been identified as the regulator of the final stages of bone formation (Nakashima et al, 2002). In similarity to Runx2, OSX also activates COL1A1 and OCN, and in a transgenic null mouse model no endochondral or intramembraneous bone formation was detected. Upstream of Runx2 the picture is less clear. A few transcription factors have been identified; Twist-1 is down-regulated for Runx2 activation, Msx2 and Bapx1 both regulate the expression of Runx2 (Huang et al, 2007). Additional studies have demonstrated the importance of signaling pathways that may act in parallel or independently of Runx2 to regulate osteoblast differentiation.

Osteoblasts also influence the differentiation of bone resorbing cells, osteoclasts. Osteoclasts derive from the monocytic / macrophage lineage and are multi-nucleated cells. The main regulatory pathway involved during osteoclast differentiation is through the receptor for activation of nuclear factor kappa B ligand (RANKL) / RANK / osteoprotegerin (OPG) pathway. Osteoblasts express RANKL and macrophage-colony stimulating factor (M-CSF), which activate a number of signaling pathways in osteoclasts. However, OPG acts as a decoy receptor for RANKL inhibiting the RANK /RANKL interaction, and in turn osteoclast differentiation. Local and systemic factors, such as parathyroid hormone (PTH) also promote osteoclast differentiation by increasing RANKL expression by osteoblasts. RANKL has also been implicated in the regulation of mature osteoclasts. OPG over-expressing transgenic mice exhibit severe osteopetrosis, impaired tooth eruption due to the lack of osteoclasts (Kong et al, 1999).

3.4 Extracellular matrix: collagenous and non-collagenous components

The organic matrix of bone is comprised of 90% collagen type I and additional non-collagenous components (Table 1), some of which have important functions in bone formation. Furthermore, the ECM is a vial source of factors that play crucial roles in cell signaling and the modulation of mineralization, such as BMPs. Most of these proteins and factors are produced locally by osteoblasts but others, like the serum proteins are synthesized elsewhere and delivered to the developing bone via the circulation.

Extracellular Matrix		
Collagenous	*Non-Collagenous*	*Enzymes*
Type I	γ-carboxyglutamic acid containing - OCN, MGP, Periostin	TNAP
Type X	Glycoproteins - ON, FN, COMP	MMPs - 1,2, 8 and 9
Type III	Sialoproteins - BSP, OPN	TIMPS - 1, 2 and 3
Type V	GAG – containing leucine rich repeat proteins - Aggrecan, Versican, DCN, BGN, FMD, LM, OSAD	
	Serum proteins - Fetuin, Albumin	

OCN -osteocalcin, *MGP* – matrix gla protein, *TNAP* – tissue non-specific alkaline phosphatase, *ON* – osteonectin, *DMP1* – dentin matrix protein 1, *FN* – fibronectin, *COMP* – thrombospondin, *MMP* – matrix metalloproteinase. *BSP* – bone sialoprotein, *OPN* – osteopontin, *TIMP* – tissue inhibitor of MMPs, *GAG* – glycosaminoglycan, *DCN* – decorin, *BGN* - biglycan, *FMD* – fibromodulin, *LM* – lumican, *OSAD* – osteoadherin

Table 1. Principal ECM-associated molecules implicated in the biomineralization process

Collagens are responsible for maintaining the structure and function of bone. In particular, fibrillar collagens, principally type I, are important in biomineralization, whereby they facilitate the formation of an ECM scaffold in which crystal nucleation occurs and subsequent crystal elongation spreads through the organized matrix. Disorders that disrupt collagen synthesis have significant effects on bone formation. In the case of OI, mutations have been identified affecting collagen type I genes, COL1A1 and COL1A2. Collagens play a crucial role during boney healing by aiding the formation of early bone spinicles that extend from the damaged / surgical site toward the center of the defect. The spinicles form the primary mineralization front associated with successful union of the surrounding bones. New bone formation associated with DO forms through the deposition of primary bone via intramembranous ossification. In a rat model of DO, studies have demonstrated that collagen type I is up-regulated ten days after osteotomy, which continues with mineralization (Fang et al, 2004).

The remaining non-collagenous proteins of bone have been implicated in the modulation and regulation of biomineralization. Most are highly anionic and have a strong ion-binding capacity. The γ-carboxyglutamic acid containing protein, OCN is known to be one of the few molecules that are truly mineralized tissue-specific (Bronckers et al, 1985). OCN acts as a regulator of mineralization through the inhibition of spontaneous mineral deposition and HAP crystal growth (Romberg et al, 1986). In DO rat models, OCN levels have been shown to correlate with successful treatment, gradually increasing from mid-activation and consolidation (Allori et al, 2008b; Fang et al, 2004). Osteonectin (ON), accounts for 15% of all non-collagenous proteins. It is proposed that ON has a role as a nucleator in collagen-mediated mineralization but also it may have a role in the inhibition of cell proliferation, modulates cell-matrix interactions, and binds and regulates HAP crystal growth (Brekken et al, 2001). A significant family of non-collagenous proteins is the small integrin-binding ligand N-linked glycoproteins (SIBLINGs). All clustered on human chromosome 4, they include bone sialoprotein (BSP) and OPN. BSP is osteoconductive, osteoinductive, promotes cell attachment, stimulates osteoblast proliferation and differentiation and importantly serves as a nucleator of mineralization (Gordon et al, 2007; Tye et al, 2003). The proteoglycan family consists of more than 30 proteins that are post-translationally modified with glycosylation or the addition of a glycosaminoglycan (GAG) chain. Small leucine-rich proteoglycans (SLRPs) have a core protein and contain one or more GAG chains including chondroitin or dermatan sulphate, heparin or keratin sulphate. Studies have shown SRLPs, in particular chondroitin sulphate-containing decorin and biglycan to bind collagen and to regulate HAP crystal growth (Sugars et al, 2003). In addition, osteoadherin (OSAD) is currently believed to be mineralized tissue-specific, with a role in inhibiting actively proliferating cells, to binding collagen and HAP (Wendel et al, 1998). Furthermore, OSAD has been found to have a similar distribution pattern as BSP in rat long bones and calvaria (Ramstad et al, 2003).

The final group of molecules that requires consideration in the ECM are enzymes, specifically tissue non-specific alkaline phosphatase (TNAP) and matrix metalloproteinases (MMPs). The current belief is that matrix mineralization is initiated through the expression of TNAP by osteoblasts. It functions to increase the relative concentration of phosphate by inactivating pyrophosphate, so that HAP becomes the main product. In disease states, such as rickets and osteomalacia, TNAP is either inactive or expressed at low levels resulting in a reduced amount of mineralization (Fedde et al, 1999). An important feature of bone formation and repair is the ability to remodel to create an environment and scaffold in which mineralization can occur. MMPs and their inhibitors, tissue inhibitors of MMPs (TIMPs) fulfill this goal and are designed to specifically degrade particular ECM components. For example, collagenases (MMP1) have been involved in fracture healing and DO, and gelatinases (MMPs 2, and 9) in osteoclastic remodeling. In addition, matrix degradation allows for growth factors and /or signaling molecules sequestered in the ECM to be released to act on early by cells (Weiss et al, 2002). MMPs also act to facilitate cell migration, influence osteogenesis and vascularization.

3.5 Growth factors and signaling molecules

The regulation of osteoblast differentiation, bone formation and turnover involves signaling molecules such as growth factors, hormones and cytokines (Table 2). These maybe secreted endogenously by local cells or absorbed from the blood. Growth factors are synthesized as biologically inactive propeptide forms and stored in the cytoplasm or ECM. They initiate their effect by binding to cell surface receptors and following intricate intracellular signaling transduction pathways to transmit signals to the nucleus, resulting in the activation of specific target genes that regulate cellular activity and or phenotype. Many act locally or systemically and affect target genes in a variety of ways; autocrine, intracrine, paracrine, juxacrine, and finally endocrine. All these mechanisms are highly regulated through a complex system of feedback loops and interactions involving other growth factors, hormones and binding proteins, as well as regulatory factors that act on extra and intracellular levels.

Principal growth factors implicated in bone formation and turnover include the transforming growth factor – β (TGF-β) family, BMPs, insulin-like growth factor (IGF), epidermal growth factor (EGF), fibroblast growth factor – 2 (FGF2), platelet-derived growth factor (PDGF) and vascular endothelial growth factor (VEGF). TGF-β isoforms 1,2 and 3 are capable of exerting the same functional activity but with slight structural differences, for example TGF-β1 has been observed at sites of osteogeneis but TGF-β's 2 and 3 at sites of chondrogenesis (Schmid et al, 1991). TGF-β's can stimulate osteoblast migration, and is a potent regulator of cell proliferation, cell differentiation and ECM maturation (Janssens et al, 2005). However, TGF-β's are unable to initiate the osteoblast and bone formation cascade at extraskeletal sites, unlike BMPs. Both TGF-β's and BMPs act via BMP receptors types I and II, and Smad 1 / 5 / 8 molecules. Phosphorylation of the Smads following binding of the BMP to the receptor causes translocation into the nucleus in a complex with Smad4, where they regulate target genes. BMPs 2, 4 and 7 are collectively known as the osteogenic BMPs as they have been shown to induce ectopic bone formation (Bragdon et al, 2011). Regulation of osteoblast differentiation results from the interaction of the complex of Smad 1 / 5 / and 8 with Smad 4 on target genes, specifically Runx2 and OSX.

Signaling Molecules		
Growth factors	*Hormones*	*Cytokines*
TGF-β	PTH	Interferon γ
BMP	Calcitonin	Interleukins 1 and 6
FGF	Estrogen	Prostaglandins E_2 and I_2
Activin A	Thyroxine	CSF
PDGF		
IGF-1		
VEGF		

TGF – transforming growth factor, *PTH* – parathyroid hormone, *BMP*- bone morphogenic protein, *FGF* – fibroblast growth factor, *CSF* –colony stimulating factor, *PDGF* –platelet derived growth factor, *IGF* – insulin growth factor, *VEGF* –vascular endothelial growth factor

Table 2. Signaling molecules involved in the regulation of bone formation and bone remodeling

A number of hormones contribute to the regulation of bone formation and turnover. Specifically of interest are PTH and calcitonin that facilitate osteoblast differentiation and calcium storage respectively (Allori et al, 2008a). PTH is secreted in response to decreased levels of calcium. Calcium release into the bloodstream following bone destruction by osteoclasts stimulates PTH and its downstream effector vitamin D3. PTH stimulates RANKL and M-CSF expression in osteoblasts but conversely inhibits OPG synthesis that in turn prevents RANKL binding to RANK. The actions of PTH and BMPs are closely linked with the activation of the Wnt signaling pathway. The Wnt / β-catenin (canonical) pathway governs osteoblast differentiation and is initiated through the formation a receptor complex, composed of Frizzled receptors and low density lipoprotein receptor-related proteins 5 and 6, on the cell surface (Westendorf et al, 2004). Activation of the canonical Wnt pathway promotes osteoblast differentiation from MSCs at the expense of adipocytes, leading to improved bone strength (Bodine et al, 2006).

3.6 Mineral composition and mechanisms of biomineralization

The major mineral component of all calcified tissues is biological apatite, a calcium phosphate that is very closely related to the geologic mineral HAP ($Ca_{10}(OH)_2(PO_4)_6$). In comparison to naturally occurring apatite, the mineral of bone differs in a number of respects, firstly biological HAP readily incorporates impurities such as CO_3^{2-}, F^-, and Na^+ into the crystal structure that are absent in pure HAP, second the theoretical calcium/phosphate ratio of pure HAP is 1.667 but this can vary from 1.5 to 1.7, leading to the term "calcium-deficient", finally a small percentage of water is present in biological HAP, making its crystallinity less than perfect. The skeleton contains 99% of the body's calcium, 35% Na^+, 60% CO_3^{2-} and 60% Mg (Boivin et al, 2003).

Biomineralization results from two stages; mineral nucleation to form HAP crystals, and subsequent HAP crystal growth, both involving the presence of the three-dimensional ECM framework. The process by which nucleation is initiated is a constant source of debate and include biomineralization foci, calcospherulites and matrix vesicles. Matrix vesicles have long been contested as sites of nucleation in bone and recent data suggested that the vesicles are present in bone but that they vary in size and the composition (Gorski, 2011). Vesicles have also been shown to be present within biomineralization foci (Huffman et al, 2007). Biomineralization foci (10-25 micron diameter) are the result of ECM-mediated nucleation. These foci are rich in acidic phosphoproteins, such as BSP and bone acidic glycoprotein -75, as well as immature collagen type I. Biomineralization foci have been detected in the periosteum of developing bones and in primary bone (Gorski et al, 2004).

3.7 Bone remodeling

Bone remodeling is a highly controlled and balanced process, ensuring the successful replacement of old bone with new through the sequential resorption by osteoclasts and subsequent bone formation by osteoblasts. Through this process bone remodeling ensures skeletal integrity throughout life. Currently, bone remodeling is considered to occur via either targeted or non-targeted remodeling (Eriksen, 2010). Non-targeted remodeling is proposed to be modulated by the osteoclasts themselves via hormones such as PTH, thyroxine and estrogen and some anti-resportive drugs like bisphosphonate. Whereas, targeted remodeling, specifically removes damaged bone and the injury of osteocytes may be the event that stimulates osteoclastic resporption. In fact, damaged osteocytes secrete M-CSF and RANKL that promote osteoclast differentiation (Kurata et al, 2006). Bone resorption occurs with the formation of the ruffled border composed of finger-shaped projections of the osteoclast membrane that mediates the process. The ruffled border forms on the surface of the bone and is only present when active resorption is occurring. This structure is also surrounded by a "clear zone", to form a microenvironment that defines the area destined to be resorbed. The mineral is dissolved through the action of an ATP-driven proton pump located in the membrane of the ruffled border. ECM, such as collagen and non-collagenous proteins are degraded through the action of MMPs, tartrate resistance acid phosphatase (TRAP) and cathespins K, B and L that are secreted by the osteoclast into the resorptive area (Bossard et al, 1996). Degraded protein components are endocytosed along the ruffled border within resorption lacunae, which are then transported to the membrane on the opposite side for release (Nesbitt et al, 1997).

4. Tissue engineering approaches and future perspectives

As highlighted above autogenous bone grafting is the most common surgical approach to treat bone defects however it does have its drawbacks including failure and rejection. There are three fundamental requirements for tissue regeneration to ensure the formation of good quality tissues that can withstand the demands of normal function: i) a source of cells to drive the regenerative process; ii) a source of growth factors and nutrients; and iii) a suitable biomaterial which can support and sustain the growth of the new tissue. However, obtaining these three components remains a challenge to tissue engineers.

4.1 Biomaterials

Several important properties, biological and physical, must be considered when developing and choosing the "ideal" biomaterial for bone grafting and regeneration procedures. The material should provide stability and possess the ability to promote osteogenesis. Physical properties include the ability to be sterilized, slow degradation rate, a high initial stiffness, a load-bearing capacity; it should be easily processed into complex-shapes and storable. Biologically, the material should be bioresorbable, biocompatible, capable of revascularization, with a highly porous and interconnected pore network to facilitate the flow and transport of nutrients and metabolic waste. In addition, the biomaterial should be either osteoconductive or osteoinductive. Osteoconductive materials act as a scaffold and the grafted material does not contribute to new bone formation *per se*. As a result an osteoconductive material enhances native bone formation in an orthotopic site. Whereas, with an osteoinductive material, it can induce bone formation in an ectopic site, in the surrounding soft tissue immediately adjacent to the grafted material by release of growth factors or other stimulatory mediators.

Four types of bone graft or substitute materials are available, autogeneous, allogenic, xenogeneic grafts and alloplastic materials. Autogeneous grafts have already been discussed, however it should be highlighted that this type of bone graft are the most osteoinductive and there is little immunological rejection. In addition, a surgical donor site is required and these tend to have a high morbidly rate. Alternatively, allogeneic grafts are widely used and occur between genetically dissimilar members of the same species. Typically frozen cancellous or freeze-dried demineralized bone is used. These grafts are both osteoconductive and osteoinductive but there is the possibility of disease transmission, loss of bone and osteogenic potential due to the treatments, and a high chance of an immunological response. Xenogeneic grafts are widely used, whereby the material is taken from the donor of another species, for example bovine. These materials are osteoconductive and do show some potential for osteoinduction but again there is the potential for disease transmission. The final type of bone graft materials are the bone fillers, synthetic or inorganic alloplastic materials that are used as bone substitutes, including HAP, β-tricalcium phosphate, polymers and bioactive glass. It remains a challenge for the bioengineers to develop a suitable biomaterial to stimulate regeneration. Modifications to provide a biomimetic surface are a particular area of study. To facilitate cell attachment is one example, and many modifications exploit cell binding motifs, such as the RGD-sequence.

4.2 Cells

In addition to the bone-building materials outlined above, the cell source has been a considerable focus in regenerative strategies. Obtaining sufficient numbers of cells with the appropriate phenotype has been a considerable challenge to the field of regenerative medicine. Ideally endogenous cells from the surrounding milieu would migrate into the defect area in the presence of a scaffold or support by cell homing. Indeed, osteoblasts may migrate from an autologous bone graft to stimulate bone formation. However, allograft, xenograft or synthetic materials lack this cell population and may require the additional application of cells. To produce bone from human stem cells could be a way to minimize the morbidity side effects. Adult stem cells have been at the forefront of regenerative medicine, in particular bone marrow-derived MSCs. However, limitations exist to using these cells as they are difficult to obtain in sufficient number due to technical problems and they are "tissue or organ-specific". Pluripotent stem cells have revolutionized stem cell research and will in all likelihood have an immense impact on the treatment of various diseases in the future. At present, groups are studying the cell lines characteristics, and developing directed differentiation strategies to the required cell type. Pluripotent stem cells, human embryonic stem cells (HSEC) or induced pluripotent stem cells (iPSCs) could overcome the obstacles hampering adult stem cell therapies. This is particularly true since derivation and culture methods have advanced considerably, and cell lines now exist that are xeno-free and could potentially be used for therapeutic purposes if the correct differentiation pathways were established.

A considerable number of studies have been performed on HESCs to induce osteogenic differentiation with many different approaches being taken (reviewed by Brown et al, 2011). Many groups have performed direct osteogenic differentiation, whereas others have taken the cells through a MSC progenitor stage prior to osteoblasts (Arpornmaeklong et al, 2009; Brown et al, 2009; Karp et al, 2006). Our own studies have shown that HESC lines differentiate along the osteogenic lineage, forming a fully mineralized bone-like matrix (Kärner et al, 2009; Kärner et al, 2007). We demonstrated the osteoblast phenotype using a large panel of extracellular matrix molecules and transcription factors (Kärner et al, 2007), and showed the dynamic gene expression of these markers (Kärner et al, 2009). In addition we characterized the deposited mineral with Fourier InfraRed spectroscopy proving that it resembled natural bone and was formed by cell-mediated mineralization. From these studies, we established a model system by which to define pluripotent stem cell osteogenic differentiation. Many technical difficulties remain be to overcome using HESCs therapeutically, as patient-matched or disease-specific HESCs will be difficult to generate, in addition to the many ethical issues to consider. One major break-through and potential solution to the problems associated with HESCs has been the derivation of iPSCs, which could eventually lead to patient-matched tissue regeneration treatments such as bone. Whether iPSCs behave in a similar manner as HESCs in terms of osteogenic differentiation remains to be determined, however the osteogenic capacity of mouse iPSCs to regenerate bone has recently been established (Bilousova et al, 2011).

Recent studies have shown that transplantation of bone grafts from a site of mesoderm tissue, such as the case of bone grafting onlay techniques, taking bone from the iliac crest to the mandible, which is neural crest derived contributes to the failure of the graft to fully integrate and regenerate bone to the standard required to withstand compressive functional processes (Chan et al, 2009; Leucht et al, 2008). These studies showed that the cell populations were not interchangeable, in that mesoderm-derived cells grafted into tibia defects produced osteoblasts but when transplanted into the mandible formed chondrocytes, and the reverse was true for neural crest-derived cells. The authors also reported that this regeneration was attributable to the homeobox gene expression pattern during embryonic development and referred to this phenomenon referred to as "positional memory" (Leucht et al, 2008). Such a finding is of considerable importance to the field of regenerative medicine, and techniques used for bone grafting procedures.

4.3 Growth factors

The ability to retain and release growth factors into the surrounding environment is crucial to ensure that cells home to the site of tissue repair and to stimulate regeneration. This has been a limiting factor to the field of tissue engineering and many obstacles remain to be overcome, including, identification of the ideal carrier, how can we sequester the growth factors to the carrier so that they remain biologically active and what is the correct dosage of the factor? Many of the growth factors are recombinantly produced, such as the BMPs and at present the amounts used for regeneration are significantly larger than those endogenously present. Adding to this is the huge cost of producing such large amounts of recombinant protein in a highly purified form.

Growth factors that are commonly used for bone regeneration include BMPs, TGF-β, FGF, VEGF, IGF, PDGF, EGF, PTH / PTH (related protein) (PTHrP) and interleukins. BMPs are involved in many developmental processes but these factors have been most widely studied in terms of bone engineering and bone replacement. Osteoblasts synthesize BMPs and sequester them in the ECM. BMPs are osteoinductive molecules and when placed ectopically they can initiate the whole pathway of bone formation from MSC differentiation to the entrapment of terminally differentiated osteoblasts as osteocytes (Wozney et al, 1988). Typically they are used in combination with many of the other factors or in combination with other family members. BMP2 and 7 have been successfully used together to facilitate boney healing (Koh et al, 2008;Ripamonti et al, 1997). The use of TGF-β's for bone regeneration has been extensively evaluated and show both stimulatory and inhibitory effects on bone formation. Despite differences in experimental setups, combined TGF-β / BMP studies show additive or synergistic effects on bone formation (Si et al, 1998; Sumner et al, 2006).

Although in many studies it has been shown that just one of these factors has been adequate to stimulate molecular and cellular events leading to regeneration, however during the natural healing process many growth factors and signaling molecules are involved simultaneously or through a cascade of events and to date it has not been possible to recapitulate this. A combination of several factors is likely to be more effective to assist boney healing.

5. Conclusions

This paper brings together clinical concepts and novel findings to the field of bone regeneration and highlights some considerations necessary when devising new strategies to treat oral-facial hard tissue defects. It is apparent from the studies described above that individuals respond differentially to stimulus; therefore future tissue engineering approaches with biomaterials, cells or growth factors will need to be tailored to the patient.

6. References

Aarden, E. M.; Burger, E. H.; Nijweide, P. J. 1994 Function of osteocytes in bone, *J Cell Biochem*, 55, 287-990730-2312.

Allori, A. C.; Sailon, A. M.; Warren, S. M. 2008b Biological basis of bone formation, remodeling, and repair-part I: biochemical signaling molecules, *Tissue Eng Part B Rev*, 14, 259-731937-3376.

Allori, A. C.; Sailon, A. M.; Warren, S. M. 2008a Biological basis of bone formation, remodeling, and repair-part II: extracellular matrix, *Tissue Eng Part B Rev*, 14, 275-831937-3376.

Arpornmaeklong, P.; Brown, S. E.; Wang, Z.; Krebsbach, P. H. 2009 Phenotypic characterization, osteoblastic differentiation, and bone regeneration capacity of human embryonic stem cell-derived mesenchymal stem cells, *Stem Cells Dev*, 18, 955-681557-8534.

Bianco, P.; Sacchetti, B.; Riminucci, M. 2011 Osteoprogenitors and the hematopoietic microenvironment, *Best Pract Res Clin Haematol*, 24, 37-471532-1924.

Bilousova, G.; Jun du, H.; King, K. B.; De Langhe, S.; Chick, W. S.; Torchia, E. C.; Chow, K. S.; Klemm, D. J.; Roop, D. R.; Majka, S. M. 2011 Osteoblasts Derived from Induced Pluripotent Stem Cells form Calcified Structures in Scaffolds Both In Vitro and In Vivo, *Stem Cells*, 29, 206-161549-4918.

Bodine, P. V.; Komm, B. S. 2006 Wnt signaling and osteoblastogenesis, *Rev Endocr Metab Disord*, 7, 33-91389-9155.

Boivin, G.; Meunier, P. J. 2003 The mineralization of bone tissue: a forgotten dimension in osteoporosis research, *Osteoporos Int*, 14 Suppl 3, S19-240937-941X.

Boyne, P. J. 1969 restoration of osseous defects in maxillofacial casualities, *J Am Dent Assoc*, 78, 767-76.

Bossard, M. J.; Tomaszek, T. A.; Thompson, S. K.; Amegadzie, B. Y.; Hanning, C. R.; Jones, C.; Kurdyla, J. T.; McNulty, D. E.; Drake, F. H.; Gowen, M.; Levy, M. A. 1996 Proteolytic activity of human osteoclast cathepsin K. Expression, purification, activation, and substrate identification, *J Biol Chem*, 271, 12517-240021-9258.

Bosshardt, D. D.; Sculean, A. 2009 Does periodontal tissue regeneration really work?, *Periodontol 2000*, 51, 208-191600-0757.

Bragdon, B.; Moseychuk, O.; Saldanha, S.; King, D.; Julian, J.; Nohe, A. 2011 Bone morphogenetic proteins: a critical review, *Cell Signal*, 23, 609-201873-3913.

Brekken, R. A.; Sage, E. H. 2001 SPARC, a matricellular protein: at the crossroads of cell-matrix communication, *Matrix Biol, 19*, 816-270945-053X.

Bronckers, A. L.; Gay, S.; Dimuzio, M. T.; Butler, W. T. 1985 Immunolocalization of gamma-carboxyglutamic acid containing proteins in developing rat bones, *Coll Relat Res, 5,* 273-810174-173X.

Brown, S. E.; Krebsbach, P. H. 2011I. Derivation of mesenchymal stem cells from human embryonic stem cellsI, In: *Embryonic Stem Cells: The Hormonal Regulation of Pluripotency and Embryogenesis*I, Atwood, C.I, pp 649-670I, InTechI, Retrieved from: http://www.intechopen.com/articles/show/title/derivation-of-mesenchymal-stem-cells-from-human-embryonic-stem-cells

Brown, S. E.; Tong, W.; Krebsbach, P. H. 2009 The derivation of mesenchymal stem cells from human embryonic stem cells, *Cells Tissues Organs, 189,* 256-601422-6421 .

Brånemark P. I.; Adell R.; Albrektsson T.; Lekholm U.; Lindström J.; Rockler B. 1984 An experimental and clinical study of osseointegrated implants penetrating the nasal cavity and maxillary sinus. *J Oral Maxillofac Surg,* 42(8):497-505.

Chan, C. K.; Chen, C. C.; Luppen, C. A.; Kim, J. B.; DeBoer, A. T.; Wei, K.; Helms, J. A.; Kuo, C. J.; Kraft, D. L.; Weissman, I. L. 2009 Endochondral ossification is required for haematopoietic stem-cell niche formation, *Nature, 457,* 490-41476-4687.

Cheung LK, Chua HDP, Hariri F, Lo J, Ow A, Zheng LW. Distraction osteogenesis. Oral and maxillofacial surgery, ed. Andersson L, Kahnberg KE, Pogrel MA, Wiley-Blackwell, 2010, chapter 48, pp. 1027-1059.

Cano J., campo J., Moreno L et al. Osteogenic alveolar distraction: A review of the literature. Oral Surg Oral Med Oral Pathol Orad <radiol Endod 101:11, 2006.

Dabirian N. and Rosén A. Implant treatment with or without bone grafting in resorbed edentulous maxillae: a two years follow-up study. Student thesis, Karolinska Institute, 2004.

Eriksen, E. F. 2010 Cellular mechanisms of bone remodeling, *Rev Endocr Metab Disord, 11,* 219-271573-2606.

Fang, T. D.; Nacamuli, R. P.; Song, H. M.; Fong, K. D.; Warren, S. M.; Salim, A.; Carano, R. A.; Filvaroff, E. H.; Longaker, M. T. 2004 Creation and characterization of a mouse model of mandibular distraction osteogenesis, *Bone, 34,* 1004-128756-3282.

Fedde, K. N.; Blair, L.; Silverstein, J.; Coburn, S. P.; Ryan, L. M.; Weinstein, R. S.; Waymire, K.; Narisawa, S.; Millan, J. L.; MacGregor, G. R.; Whyte, M. P. 1999 Alkaline phosphatase knock-out mice recapitulate the metabolic and skeletal defects of infantile hypophosphatasia, *J Bone Miner Res, 14,* 2015-260884-0431.

Giannoudis, P. V.; Dinopoulos, H.; Tsiridis, E. 2005 Bone substitutes: an update, *Injury, 36* Suppl 3, S20-70020-1383.

Gordon, J. A.; Tye, C. E.; Sampaio, A. V.; Underhill, T. M.; Hunter, G. K.; Goldberg, H. A. 2007 Bone sialoprotein expression enhances osteoblast differentiation and matrix mineralization in vitro, *Bone, 41,* 462-738756-3282.

Gorski, J. P. 2011 Biomineralization of bone: a fresh view of the roles of non-collagenous proteins, *Front Biosci, 17,* 2598-6211093-4715.

Gorski, J. P.; Wang, A.; Lovitch, D.; Law, D.; Powell, K.; Midura, R. J. 2004 Extracellular bone acidic glycoprotein-75 defines condensed mesenchyme regions to be mineralized and localizes with bone sialoprotein during intramembranous bone formation, *J Biol Chem, 279,* 25455-630021-9258.

Harada, H.; Tagashira, S.; Fujiwara, M.; Ogawa, S.; Katsumata, T.; Yamaguchi, A.; Komori, T.; Nakatsuka, M. 1999 Cbfa1 isoforms exert functional differences in osteoblast differentiation, *J Biol Chem, 274*, 6972-80021-9258.

Huang, W.; Yang, S.; Shao, J.; Li, Y. P. 2007 Signaling and transcriptional regulation in osteoblast commitment and differentiation, *Front Biosci, 12*, 3068-921093-4715.

Huffman, N. T.; Keightley, J. A.; Chaoying, C.; Midura, R. J.; Lovitch, D.; Veno, P. A.; Dallas, S. L.; Gorski, J. P. 2007 Association of specific proteolytic processing of bone sialoprotein and bone acidic glycoprotein-75 with mineralization within biomineralization foci, *J Biol Chem, 282*, 26002-130021-9258.

Janssens, K.; ten Dijke, P.; Janssens, S.; Van Hul, W. 2005 Transforming growth factor-beta1 to the bone, *Endocr Rev, 26*, 743-740163-769X.

Kahnberg KE. Treatment of bone deficient ridges in implant rehabilitation. Oral and maxillofacial surgery, ed. Andersson L, Kahnberg KE, Pogrel MA, Wiley-Blackwell, 2010, chapter 24, pp. 405-414.

Krekmanow L., Kahn M., Rangert B, et al. tilting of posterior mandibular and maxillary implants for improved prothesis support. Int J Oral Maxillofac Implants 15:405, 2000.

Kärner, E.; Backesjo, C. M.; Cedervall, J.; Sugars, R. V.; Ahrlund-Richter, L.; Wendel, M. 2009 Dynamics of gene expression during bone matrix formation in osteogenic cultures derived from human embryonic stem cells in vitro, *Biochim Biophys Acta, 1790*, 110-80006-3002.

Kärner, E.; Unger, C.; Sloan, A. J.; Ahrlund-Richter, L.; Sugars, R. V.; Wendel, M. 2007 Bone matrix formation in osteogenic cultures derived from human embryonic stem cells in vitro, *Stem Cells Dev, 16*, 39-521547-3287.

Karp, J. M.; Ferreira, L. S.; Khademhosseini, A.; Kwon, A. H.; Yeh, J.; Langer, R. S. 2006 Cultivation of human embryonic stem cells without the embryoid body step enhances osteogenesis in vitro, *Stem Cells, 24*, 835-431066-5099.

Koh, J. T.; Zhao, Z.; Wang, Z.; Lewis, I. S.; Krebsbach, P. H.; Franceschi, R. T. 2008 Combinatorial gene therapy with BMP2/7 enhances cranial bone regeneration, *J Dent Res, 87*, 845-90022-0345.

Komori, T.; Yagi, H.; Nomura, S.; Yamaguchi, A.; Sasaki, K.; Deguchi, K.; Shimizu, Y.; Bronson, R. T.; Gao, Y. H.; Inada, M.; Sato, M.; Okamoto, R.; Kitamura, Y.; Yoshiki, S.; Kishimoto, T. 1997 Targeted disruption of Cbfa1 results in a complete lack of bone formation owing to maturational arrest of osteoblasts, *Cell, 89*, 755-640092-8674.

Kong, Y. Y.; Feige, U.; Sarosi, I.; Bolon, B.; Tafuri, A.; Morony, S.; Capparelli, C.; Li, J.; Elliott, R.; McCabe, S.; Wong, T.; Campagnuolo, G.; Moran, E.; Bogoch, E. R.; Van, G.; Nguyen, L. T.; Ohashi, P. S.; Lacey, D. L.; Fish, E.; Boyle, W. J.; Penninger, J. M. 1999 Activated T cells regulate bone loss and joint destruction in adjuvant arthritis through osteoprotegerin ligand, *Nature, 402*, 304-90028-0836.

Kurata, K.; Heino, T. J.; Higaki, H.; Vaananen, H. K. 2006 Bone marrow cell differentiation induced by mechanically damaged osteocytes in 3D gel-embedded culture, *J Bone Miner Res, 21*, 616-250884-0431.

Kurt G., Altug-Atac AT., Atac MS., Karasu HA. Stability of surgically assisted rapid maxillary expansion and orthopedic maxillary expansion after 3 years follow-up. Angle orthodontist, 80;4:613-619, 2010.

Leucht, P.; Kim, J. B.; Amasha, R.; James, A. W.; Girod, S.; Helms, J. A. 2008 Embryonic origin and Hox status determine progenitor cell fate during adult bone regeneration, *Development, 135*, 2845-540950-1991.

Marie, P. J. 2008 Transcription factors controlling osteoblastogenesis, *Arch Biochem Biophys, 473*, 98-1051096-0384.

Maiorana C. Biomaterials for bone replacement in implant surgery. Oral and maxillofacial surgery, ed. Andersson L, Kahnberg KE, Pogrel MA, Wiley-Blackwell, 2010, chapter 26, pp. 425-437.

Martin, E.; Shapiro, J. R. 2007 Osteogenesis imperfecta:epidemiology and pathophysiology, *Curr Osteoporos Rep, 5*, 91-71544-1873.

Mattson T., Köndell PÅ., Gynther G., et al. Implant treatment without bone grafting in severely resorbed edentulous maxillae. J Oral Maxillofac Surg 57:281, 1999.

Nakashima, K.; Zhou, X.; Kunkel, G.; Zhang, Z.; Deng, J. M.; Behringer, R. R.; de Crombrugghe, B. 2002 The novel zinc finger-containing transcription factor osterix is required for osteoblast differentiation and bone formation, *Cell, 108*, 17-290092-8674.

Nesbitt, S. A.; Horton, M. A. 1997 Trafficking of matrix collagens through bone-resorbing osteoclasts, *Science, 276*, 266-90036-8075.

Nyström E., Ahlqvist J., Kahnberg KE. 10-years follow-up of onlay bone grafts and implants in severely resorbed maxillae. Int J Oral Maxillofac Surg 33:258, 2004.

Ramstad, V. E.; Franzen, A.; Heinegard, D.; Wendel, M.; Reinholt, F. P. 2003 Ultrastructural distribution of osteoadherin in rat bone shows a pattern similar to that of bone sialoprotein, *Calcif Tissue Int, 72*, 57-640171-967X.

Ripamonti, U.; Duneas, N.; Van Den Heever, B.; Bosch, C.; Crooks, J. 1997 Recombinant transforming growth factor-beta1 induces endochondral bone in the baboon and synergizes with recombinant osteogenic protein-1 (bone morphogenetic protein-7) to initiate rapid bone formation, *J Bone Miner Res, 12*, 1584-950884-0431.

Romberg, R. W.; Werness, P. G.; Riggs, B. L.; Mann, K. G. 1986 Inhibition of hydroxyapatite crystal growth by bone-specific and other calcium-binding proteins, *Biochemistry, 25*, 1176-800006-2960.

Rosén A., Gynther G. Implant treatment without bone grafting in severely resorbed edentulous maxillas: A long-term follow up study. J Oral Maxillofac Surg 65:1010-1016, 2007.

Rosén A., Modig M., Larson O. Orthognathic bimaxillary surgery in two patients with osteogenesis imperfecta and a review of the literature. Int J Oral Maxillofac Surg 2011, Aug; 40(8):866-73. Epub 2011 Apr 3.

Rosén A., Kruger Weiner C. Three years follow up of distraction osteogenesis treatment in two patient with frontal open bite and a review of the literature. In manuscript 2011.

Saulacic N., Zix J., Iizuka T. Complication rates and associated factors in alveolar distraction osteogenesis: a comprehensive review. Int J Oral Maxillofac Surg 2009, 38(3):210-7. Epub 2009 Feb 14.

Schmid, P.; Cox, D.; Bilbe, G.; Maier, R.; McMaster, G. K. 1991 Differential expression of TGF beta 1, beta 2 and beta 3 genes during mouse embryogenesis, *Development, 111*, 117-300950-1991.

Si, X.; Jin, Y.; Yang, L. 1998 Induction of new bone by ceramic bovine bone with recombinant human bone morphogenetic protein 2 and transforming growth factor beta, *Int J Oral Maxillofac Surg*, *27*, 310-40901-5027.

Sugars, R. V.; Milan, A. M.; Brown, J. O.; Waddington, R. J.; Hall, R. C.; Embery, G. 2003 Molecular interaction of recombinant decorin and biglycan with type I collagen influences crystal growth, *Connect Tissue Res*, *44 Suppl 1*, 189-950300-8207.

Sumner, D. R.; Turner, T. M.; Urban, R. M.; Virdi, A. S.; Inoue, N. 2006 Additive enhancement of implant fixation following combined treatment with rhTGF-beta2 and rhBMP-2 in a canine model, *J Bone Joint Surg Am*, *88*, 806-170021-9355.

Takeda, S.; Bonnamy, J. P.; Owen, M. J.; Ducy, P.; Karsenty, G. 2001 Continuous expression of Cbfa1 in nonhypertrophic chondrocytes uncovers its ability to induce hypertrophic chondrocyte differentiation and partially rescues Cbfa1-deficient mice, *Genes Dev*, *15*, 467-810890-9369.

Triplett, R. G.; Schow S. R.; Laskin D. M. 2000 Oral and maxillofacial surgery advances in implant dentistry, *Int J Oral Maxillofac Surg 15(1)*, 47-55.

Tye, C. E.; Rattray, K. R.; Warner, K. J.; Gordon, J. A.; Sodek, J.; Hunter, G. K.; Goldberg, H. A. 2003 Delineation of the hydroxyapatite-nucleating domains of bone sialoprotein, *J Biol Chem*, *278*, 7949-550021-9258.

Weiss, S.; Baumgart, R.; Jochum, M.; Strasburger, C. J.; Bidlingmaier, M. 2002 Systemic regulation of distraction osteogenesis: a cascade of biochemical factors, *J Bone Miner Res*, *17*, 1280-90884-0431.

Wendel, M.; Sommarin, Y.; Heinegard, D. 1998 Bone matrix proteins: isolation and characterization of a novel cell-binding keratan sulfate proteoglycan (osteoadherin) from bovine bone, *J Cell Biol*, *141*, 839-470021-9525.

Westendorf, J. J.; Kahler, R. A.; Schroeder, T. M. 2004 Wnt signaling in osteoblasts and bone diseases, *Gene*, *341*, 19-390378-1119.

Wikesjsö, U.; Polimeni, G.; Xiropadidis, A.; Stravropoulos, A. *Peridontal wound healing/regeneration*; Quintessence: London, 2010.

Wozney, J. M.; Rosen, V.; Celeste, A. J.; Mitsock, L. M.; Whitters, M. J.; Kriz, R. W.; Hewick, R. M.; Wang, E. A. 1988 Novel regulators of bone formation: molecular clones and activities, *Science*, *242*, 1528-340036-8075.

Permissions

The contributors of this book come from diverse backgrounds, making this book a truly international effort. This book will bring forth new frontiers with its revolutionizing research information and detailed analysis of the nascent developments around the world.

We would like to thank Alessandro Rozim Zorzi, MD, MSc and João Batista de Miranda, MD, PhD, for lending their expertise to make the book truly unique. They have played a crucial role in the development of this book. Without their invaluable contribution this book wouldn't have been possible. They have made vital efforts to compile up to date information on the varied aspects of this subject to make this book a valuable addition to the collection of many professionals and students.

This book was conceptualized with the vision of imparting up-to-date information and advanced data in this field. To ensure the same, a matchless editorial board was set up. Every individual on the board went through rigorous rounds of assessment to prove their worth. After which they invested a large part of their time researching and compiling the most relevant data for our readers. Conferences and sessions were held from time to time between the editorial board and the contributing authors to present the data in the most comprehensible form. The editorial team has worked tirelessly to provide valuable and valid information to help people across the globe.

Every chapter published in this book has been scrutinized by our experts. Their significance has been extensively debated. The topics covered herein carry significant findings which will fuel the growth of the discipline. They may even be implemented as practical applications or may be referred to as a beginning point for another development. Chapters in this book were first published by InTech; hereby published with permission under the Creative Commons Attribution License or equivalent.

The editorial board has been involved in producing this book since its inception. They have spent rigorous hours researching and exploring the diverse topics which have resulted in the successful publishing of this book. They have passed on their knowledge of decades through this book. To expedite this challenging task, the publisher supported the team at every step. A small team of assistant editors was also appointed to further simplify the editing procedure and attain best results for the readers.

Our editorial team has been hand-picked from every corner of the world. Their multi-ethnicity adds dynamic inputs to the discussions which result in innovative outcomes. These outcomes are then further discussed with the researchers and contributors who give their valuable feedback and opinion regarding the same. The feedback is then collaborated with the researches and they are edited in a comprehensive manner to aid the understanding of the subject.

Apart from the editorial board, the designing team has also invested a significant amount of their time in understanding the subject and creating the most relevant covers. They scrutinized every image to scout for the most suitable representation of the subject and create an appropriate cover for the book.

The publishing team has been involved in this book since its early stages. They were actively engaged in every process, be it collecting the data, connecting with the contributors or procuring relevant information. The team has been an ardent support to the editorial, designing and production team. Their endless efforts to recruit the best for this project, has resulted in the accomplishment of this book. They are a veteran in the field of academics and their pool of knowledge is as vast as their experience in printing. Their expertise and guidance has proved useful at every step. Their uncompromising quality standards have made this book an exceptional effort. Their encouragement from time to time has been an inspiration for everyone.

The publisher and the editorial board hope that this book will prove to be a valuable piece of knowledge for researchers, students, practitioners and scholars across the globe.

List of Contributors

Alessandro Rozim Zorzi and João Batista de Miranda
Campinas State University - UNICAMP, Brazil

Nguyen Ngoc Hung
Hanoi Medial University, Military Academy of Medicine, Pediatric Orthopaedic Department
National Hospital of Pediatrics, Dong Da District, Ha Noi, Vietnam

Olivier Cornu
Orthopaedic and Trauma Department, Cliniques Universitaires St-Luc, Université Catholique
de Louvain, Brussels, Belgium

R. Adani
Hand and Microsurgery Department, Policlinico GB Rossi, Azienda Ospedaliera Universitaria
Verona,Verona, Italy

L. Tarallo and R. Mugnai
Department of Orthopaedic Surgery, University of Modena and Reggio Emilia, Policlinico
di Modena, Modena, Italy

Fernando Baldy dos Reis
Orthopedics and Traumatology Department, Universidade Federal de São Paulo (Unifesp),
São Paulo, Brazil

Jean Klay Santos Machado
Porto Dias and Adventista de Belém Hospitals, Pará, Brazil

Sudhir Babhulkar
Indira Gandhi Medical College, Nagpur, Sushrut Hosp, Research Centre & PGI, Nagpur,
India

Dror Paley
Paley Institute, St. Mary's Hospital, West Palm Beach, Florida, USA

Deng Lei, Ma Zhanzhong, Yang Huaikuo, Xue Lei and Yang Gongbo
Orthopaedic Department, Beijing XiYuan Hospital, China Academy of Chinese Medical
Science, China

Majid Reza Farrokhi and Golnaz Yadollahi Khales
Shiraz Neurosciences Research Center, Shiraz University of Medical Sciences, Shiraz, Iran

Bernhard Pommer, Werner Zechner and Georg Watzek
Department of Oral Surgery, Vienna Medical University, Austria

Richard Palmer
Department of Restorative Dentistry, King's College London, UK

Annika Rosén and Rachael Sugars
Div of Oral and Maxillofacial Surgery and the Craniofacial Stem Cell Biology Group, Div of Oral Biology, Dept. of Dental Medicine, Karolinska Institutet, Huddinge, Sweden

Printed in the USA
CPSIA information can be obtained
at www.ICGtesting.com
JSHW011408221024
72173JS00003B/462